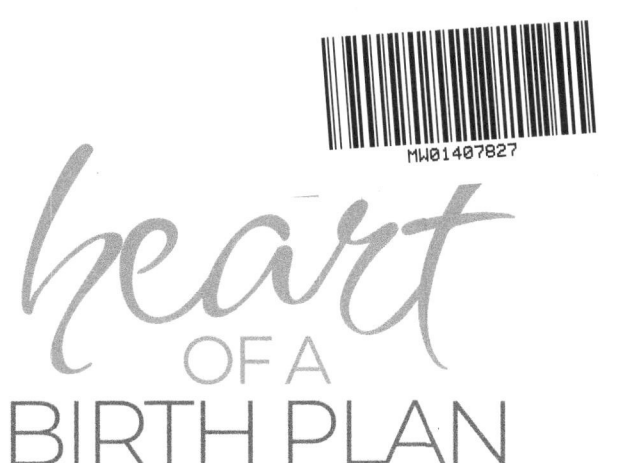

heart OF A BIRTH PLAN

THE heart OF A BIRTH PLAN

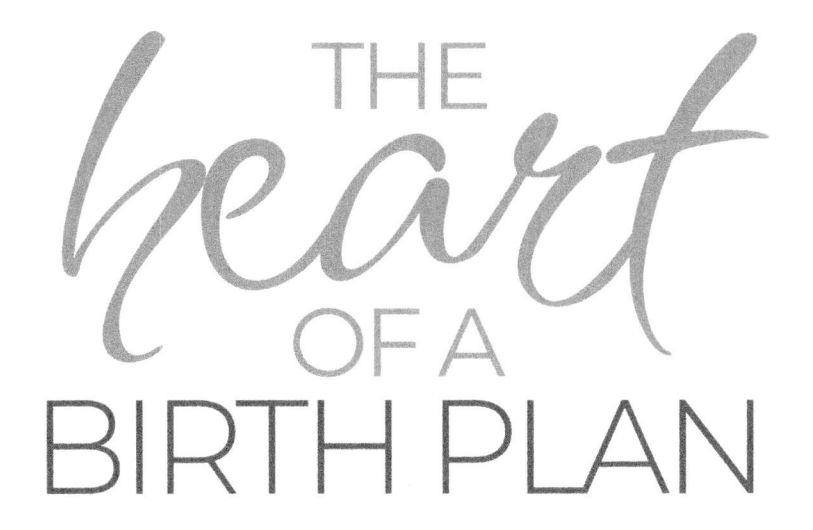

A Labor Nurse's Guide to the Best Hospital Birth Experience and How Biblical Concepts Come Alive in the Process of Labor, Birth, and New Life

MARIA MAHER, RN

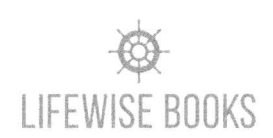

LIFEWISE BOOKS

THE HEART OF A BIRTH PLAN

A Labor Nurse's Guide to the Best Hospital Birth Experience and How Biblical Concepts Come Alive in the Process of Labor, Birth, and New Life

BY MARIA MAHER, RN

Copyright © 2022 Maria Maher, BSN; RNC-EFM. All rights reserved. Except for brief quotations for review purposes, no part of this book may be reproduced in any form without prior written permission from the author.

All verses ESV unless otherwise noted.

Scriptures marked ESV are taken from the THE HOLY BIBLE, ENGLISH STANDARD VERSION (ESV): Scriptures taken from THE HOLY BIBLE, ENGLISH STANDARD VERSION ® Copyright© 2001 by Crossway, a publishing ministry of Good News Publishers. Used by permission.

Scriptures marked NIV are taken from the NEW INTERNATIONAL VERSION (NIV): Scripture taken from THE HOLY BIBLE, NEW INTERNATIONAL VERSION ®. Copyright© 1973, 1978, 1984, 2011 by Biblica, Inc.™. Used by permission of Zondervan

PUBLISHED BY:

LIFEWISE BOOKS
PO BOX 1072
Pinehurst, TX 77362
LifeWiseBooks.com

To contact the author: mariamaher.com

ISBN (Print): 978-1-952247-74-3
ISBN (Ebook): 978-1-952247-75-0

DEDICATION

This writing is dedicated to all of the pregnant ladies who became mothers in front of my eyes over the years as a hospital labor nurse. You are the reason for my work and have taught me so much. This is also for the mothers in postpartum who challenged me by being honest about their labor experience and the pains of the unexpected. You led me to search for more and helped me to make the spiritual connection that made this book possible.

SPECIAL ACKNOWLEDGMENTS AND THANKS

I want to thank all the nurses I have worked with over the years, especially on the night shift. The night shift years of my career were so very special to me. You all have invested in me, taught me, laughed with me, corrected me, and were my tribe. I will forever remember the 3:00 a.m. stories and camaraderie we shared while teaming up to care for these pregnant ladies. The labor nurses I have known over the years have put on their scrubs to care for these mothers while "putting off" their own life struggles, marriages, motherhood, and comfort all for the direct patient care of laboring mothers. I applaud you. You are all amazing.

I want to thank my husband and a few very special people who encouraged me on my writing journey. God brought different people into my path throughout my time contemplating and writing this book. I am thankful for the writers who spoke into the writing aspect of my journey, the nurses who encouraged my train of thought, and my Bible study ladies over time who encouraged me to trust God through this project. My husband has had a front-row seat for all the doubts and fear associated with this work and has always encouraged me to reach for obedience in what I believed God had for me with this writing. Myron, I love you and appreciate you more than you know. Thank you for believing in my words.

CONTENTS

INTRODUCTION
Getting to the Heart of a Birth Plan ... 1

   CHAPTER ONE
   Preparing for a Hospital Birth in Three Rhythms: Mind, Nurse, and Spirit ... 7

   CHAPTER TWO
   Hospital Orientation: Realistic Expectations about Our Birth Setting ... 25

   CHAPTER THREE
   An Orientation to Your Nurse ... 59

   CHAPTER FOUR
   Can We Talk Comfortably About Being Uncomfortable? ... 83

   CHAPTER FIVE
   Listening Between the Heartbeats and Hearing Your Spiritual Truth ... 101

   CHAPTER SIX
   Physical Birth as a Spiritual Picture ... 125

ABCS OF SALVATION ... 143

ABOUT THE AUTHOR ... 145

ENDNOTES ... 147

introduction
GETTING TO THE HEART OF A BIRTH PLAN

Hello, reader! Thank you for your curiosity as to what exactly *is* the "heart of a birth plan." When we are addressing something as common as labor and birth, it is not surprising that many opinions exist on the subject. I know many have gone before me in writing advice to the pregnant population of expectant mothers. But when I think about what has served the patients in the hospital the most, it has to do with the heart. The heart of the matter is how you view your own birth story. What I have found is who you believe to be the author of it will play a huge role in how you see yourself in your own story of pregnancy and birth.

I want to tell you a little bit of who I am and how I came to write this book. I am a very ordinary woman, who happens to be a labor and delivery nurse. I also happen to be a Christian and have been imperfectly following the Lord for twenty years. I am a constant learner and have definitely been known as the "quizmeister" by a few different people mentoring me in the hospital over the years.

I love digging and discovering the "why" of what we do in the hospital. I love the discipline of labor and delivery because there is always an opportunity for learning and seeing something new. You never actually "know it all." I have also had the same experience with the Bible. No matter how long I've been reading it, there's always new insight, new learning that comes with the text. My journey to writing this book converges in a way that I began to see biblical truths in my everyday job of being with women during their labor and birth.

I firmly believe God uses ordinary things (and often ordinary people) to show spiritual truths in a way that we can understand. I knew in the New Testament of the Bible, He uses examples of fishing for the fishermen, shepherd illustrations for those who knew sheep, planting/harvesting illustrations for the agrarian mindset, and multiple parables taken right out of everyday life for the benefit of those listening.

So, was there a hidden spiritual truth tucked away in the discipline of delivering babies and laboring mothers? I started to look and listen. Listening to laboring mothers and the mothers in postpartum, I began seeing patterns emerge from the discipline of childbearing. Curiosity opened my senses to pay attention to what God might be showing me every day through the common worldly experience of labor, birth, and new life.

I started to see a spiritual element of struggle with birth. Some women are doing well with their birth, and some are struggling during labor and birth more than others. I have a heart to speak into this spiritual struggle as a writer and a nurse. As a nurse, I find myself speaking to my patients about releasing control and embracing the true situation of their birth story. I know other nurses are at the bedside holding the hands of their patients and speaking truths to their patients, which may be, unbeknownst to them, biblical concepts.

Physical pain needs to be addressed physically in tangible ways, whether it's position changes or medications. But the spiritual angst of the overwhelming number of women coming to the birth room with anxiety, fear, and a gripping need for control needs to be addressed, but maybe in a new way.

I know there is a lot of writing out there for pregnant mothers making promises. Some writings are to inform a patient on pain-control strategies or education offerings of the physicality of birth, literally describing the physiology of how the baby will come out of your body. Some offerings are how to take control in the birth room to empower yourself in your birth. Others are offerings giving recipes of how to refuse or accept interventions in the hospital environment in order to have the best births. Mine is none of these. My offering here is simply my best advice for the heart of a hospital laboring mother.

Hospital births are undervalued and are often seen by common writings as something to fear or the place where empowering birth plans go to die. I want to share with the women who are having hospital-style births as to how they can prepare for birth with a biblical mindset. I want to show you how to see yourself in your own birth story without emotional birth trauma, false guilt, or confusion when you hold that beautiful baby in postpartum. I want to revive old truths that have stood the test of time in God's Holy Word. I want to show the modern woman of today how old truths are alive and active and will be present inside the birth room.

I believe a positive birthing experience should be had by all women, not only women who have natural unmedicated births, or women whose birth plans become their reality, but all women. The hospital in general is a place where people with problems go. That is true in labor and delivery as well. We genuinely have a population of people who need a hospital-style birth due to their specific diagnosis or pregnancy situation. They, too, deserve to perceive their birth experience as positive, not less than someone else.

Understanding what to expect in a hospital can go a long way toward a positive birth experience. In fact, I believe unmet expectations contribute profoundly to you not seeing your hospital experience as fulfilling. It is with postpartum in mind, working with women recovering from their birth after delivery, that I have come to see we need to prepare women for hospital birth in three rhythms: mind, nurse, and spirit.

Understanding how the hospital functions and learning its predictable sequence of care will help you to have realistic expectations. Having realistic expectations is the "mind" element and will help to relieve fear as you will be able to discern where you are in the process of labor and birth.

I wanted to write this book to inform, always having the plan to prepare a woman for a hospital birth but addressing areas not commonly written about or informed of in prenatal education. I want to give you a peek behind the curtain of a hospital environment and introduce you to the team who works there. I have found it is a team of people very different from what was told to me during my birthing education when I was pregnant and not a nurse. I want to show you the truths of what I have learned about the hospital setting itself.

The second rhythm is understanding your nurse as your gifted guide through your hospital experience and how to value this resource so you can improve your hospital experience. Understanding the role and impact of your assigned nurse is paramount to a positive hospital birth experience. This is the most overlooked aspect of preparing a mother for hospital life and a missed opportunity for hospitals to prepare patients prenatally. I wish every pregnant woman could get inside the mind of a labor nurse about their particular situation and could understand how important relating to your nurse will be for your whole experience. Most patients who come to the hospital don't really even know what we do.

Now that you are reading this book, you will come to the hospital with knowledge of the setting itself and what the role of the nurse is who will be assigned to you. It will make a huge difference, trust me. If you did nothing else, learning about the hospital environment and what to expect coupled with the knowledge of how to value your labor nurse will dramatically improve your hospital experience as a birthing mom.

But when addressing how to have a better hospital birth, covering the mind and the nurse is straightforward. Speaking into spiritual matters of the heart is more difficult, yet the core issue. It will help you the most, not only with your birth but assigning it meaning. The spiritual element is the true heart of a birth plan. But everyone who is trying to have a better hospital birth may be at a different place spiritually.

I have imagined the faces of the multicultural, multifaith demographics of the population I serve at my hospital. There are so many women of different faiths and beliefs whom I serve at my location, and I tried to see their faces as I wrote this book, making efforts to serve them in my writing to truly have a better hospital birth, while telling the truth about the heart of the matter.

Truth be told, I have written this book in a way that WILL help someone of any faith have a better hospital experience. But unapologetically, I have written with the Bible as my source of truth when it comes to the spiritual lessons I have learned and feel compelled to share. Trying to remove the biblical connection is gutting the entire heart of the book and removing what moved me to write it in the first place. That's why I couldn't remove it. God is not done showing us new things, and the spiritual element can soothe the parts of your story that need a different kind of answer.

I pray this will help you see your birth differently, and I truly hope it helps you to hold your precious little one in postpartum with a heart full of peace and eyes to survey the hospital scene with a new perception. This book is the attempt from an ordinary woman to share the glory of an extraordinary God through a common physical phenomenon happening all over the world: birth.

With surrendered spirit,

Maria Maher

BSN; RNC-EFM

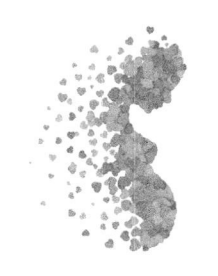

chapter one
PREPARING FOR A HOSPITAL BIRTH IN THREE RHYTHMS: MIND, NURSE, AND SPIRIT

As a nurse, I get my patient assignment for the day. Today, I am working postpartum, helping moms who have already delivered their babies and are trying to establish bonding and feeding routines. I walk into my first postpartum room and hear the patient tell me she's disappointed she got an epidural. She wasn't planning on it, but the contractions just "hurt too much." It somehow wasn't what she was expecting. She's holding this beautiful baby, but yet is sad talking about her birth, and there's an aura of defeat. I comfort her and move on.

Next room, a mother is coping with her baby being in the neonatal intensive care unit (NICU). Her labor had unforeseen problems, and her baby needed extra care after delivery. She is tearful as I comfort her and help her learn to use the breast pump. She's feeling unprepared for this situation because it wasn't what she was expecting.

In the next room is a couple doting over their baby, sharing pictures and face-timing with family, so proud of their baby. When I ask about her labor experience, she says, "I almost delivered in the car! We barely made it to the hospital!" The mom and dad both laugh as they tell me their birth story and how crazy different it was from what they were planning, which was a pain-free epidural birth.

My next patient is an experienced mom. She tells me how her others were much easier than this one. This baby had a harder labor and for some reason is having a hard time nursing. Her others didn't. It just wasn't what she was expecting and somehow different from her other births.

Now, I'm not the sharpest tool in the shed, but after years of working both labor and postpartum, I have heard the ringing sentiment of, "It wasn't what I was expecting!" almost every night I work a postpartum assignment. It looks different for different situations, and ladies will describe it differently, but it is always similar in tone.

Sometimes it sounds like this:

> *"I didn't know breastfeeding was so hard."*
>
> *"I didn't know I would bleed this much...is this normal?"*
>
> *"I never thought I would be here for three days trying to have my baby."*
>
> *"I got an epidural because I just wasn't tough enough I guess."*

"Is it normal for the baby to cry this much?"

"Is my baby getting enough when I'm nursing? It's as if they want to be at the breast all the time."

It honestly seems like some sort of postpartum mantra. If you really ask about someone's birth story, they love to tell you. But if you follow it with, "Was it what you were expecting?" you usually will get some sort of reason for why it wasn't.

So true! In fact, isn't life in general that way? How many times have you gone into a situation expecting one thing and being surprised in the middle left you confused or frustrated on the back end? Have you ever started something new, like getting married or starting a school program or getting a puppy, only to find out there's so much more you didn't even know existed? But here you are in this new thing, committed, but trying to figure out the best way to move forward in it.

OUR FENWAY

I have a dog who has been my example of this phenomenon. I was in love with a sweet little dog named Wrigley. He was the best dog in the west. He was my little fat buddy. He loved to lay everywhere and would begrudgingly take a short walk daily. I was introduced to a beautiful Australian shepherd my dog loved. They played and seemed like fast friends. I had no idea of what to expect by getting an Aussie, but we adopted her and named her Fenway.

The energy level was off the charts, and I found myself in unfamiliar territory of my home being destroyed (chewed into oblivion), a dog who couldn't walk normally on a leash, didn't like visitors, and howled if she was put in the backyard. It was a complete shock. But we were committed and worked with her. Imperfectly, we moved forward with our new dog and our new reality.

Soon after, my dog Wrigley passed away, and my new reality was an Aussie named Fenway who really, really needed special attention! Of course, she trusted us by this point, and we had already bonded with her as part of our family. So, the answer was to try to learn about my Aussie and accept the things about her that truly were not a fit originally. By changing our expectations, we were able to embrace the positives of who my Aussie truly is, and honor her breed.

Truly, the greatest was when we were able to take a road trip to my mother-in-law's property in Missouri and see her unleashed on forty-seven acres with cows! My dog loved to be out there with the cows and somehow had amazing recall skills out there on all that land! Now, I know to expect that every morning my dog will crawl up on my chest, and as soon as I open my eyes, I know she wants to "go" as we call it. My day will proceed with normality if I exercise Fenway first thing in the morning. I've come to expect it, and I know she needs it.

We are now looking into herding lessons close to our home because it's a beautiful thing to embrace that which she was created to be, not what I wanted her to be. Changing my expectations to be more realistic of what an Aussie truly is like is creating a more positive perception of my dog. I'm seeing less "wrong" with *her* and more of what was wrong with *my* unrealistic expectations. And it's changing how I see my dog.

Expecting a baby is like that. It's this wonderful new thing that is always built up with such grandeur, and rightfully so. But the actual labor and delivery of this sweet baby will often set us on a course into the unexpected. It is in the uncharted waters of the hospital environment during our birth that we will be changed into a mother of a new life, some for the first time. Change is always the beginning of something new, and sometimes with beginning something new, we will be changed in the process. Changing what we expect out of a hospital birth just may change our perceptions enough to appreciate it for what it is made to be, maybe not what we wanted it to be.

HOSPITAL BREED

Hospitals get a bad rap for birthing experiences, and it really need not be so. Hospitals are set up for a certain type of delivery style; they are a certain breed. That delivery style is caring for those who have problems or diagnoses with pregnancy who *will* actually need intervention. Normal healthy moms who have a hospital environment delivery will be part of the hospital experience, as it was set up to be. They may not need the interventions that others with diagnoses do but, nevertheless, are going to be part of the delivery environment in the same sequence of care as every other admitted labor patient.

For example, as obesity, hypertension, and diabetes climb in our general population, we see higher numbers of pregnant moms with these diagnoses too. A pregnant mom with this situation can expect more continuous fetal monitoring, lab testing, blood sugars, and medications as part of their labor and delivery. A healthy mom giving birth in this setting will have the same precautions as the higher risk patient, such as having an IV placed and fetal monitoring of her baby, but will require less intervention. Maybe the healthy mom will have her IV placed but not running with IV fluids or maybe monitoring for shorter periods of time with some periods off the monitor.

In this hospital breed of birth setting, there will still be hospital rules. There is still a hierarchy of professionals with different scopes of practice who will function within the bounds of their medical licenses. Additionally, there will be all the hospital "processes" that exist in this discipline. For example, every labor patient will have vitals taken. If you are a healthy lady, it may look like vitals every four hours vs. the high-risk patient on intervention medications for blood pressures who may need vitals every ten minutes until they are stabilized. But everyone gets vitals in the hospital. There are many hospital constants like this that are true for everyone, yet different from person to person.

PATIENT EXPECTATIONS

Hospital life is hospital life and is going to remain constant in this breed of birth setting. There is a disconnect between the hospital culture and patient expectations that can cause unwanted friction in patient care sometimes. Most of our time spent as bedside nurses is spent on educating women about what to expect next, and what it will look like moving forward through the process of a hospital delivery and a postpartum experience.

I have found that if a patient's expectations are managed well, then their experience as a whole is perceived better. I have a passion to help women feel better in postpartum about their overall hospital experience. No woman deserves to feel guilty or ashamed because they opted for pain control or had a cesarean section. Each woman deserves to heal from their birth, while looking at their beautiful baby, appreciating their experience as a whole.

I want to change how you see yourself in your own birth story. I want you to feel better about knowing what to expect about the "breed" of hospital birth and what it was meant to be. I want you to see yourself differently in your story, and I believe the way to do that is to appreciate the truths of the hospital environment and use them to your advantage. I believe there are amazing resources available to a patient having a hospital birth, and they are called nurses.

Your assigned labor nurse is the most undervalued resource for you during your time in the hospital. I want to show you how she can be of value to your overall experience. I want to peel back the curtain on the people you will meet as your nurses during your stay and introduce you to them. Your nurse can entirely "make" your birthing experience, and in prenatal education, we don't really even discuss their value to patients. From what I've seen, patients come into the hospital thinking the doctor is somehow going to be with them, and they are surprised to see more nurses than anything else during their stay.

Most education I do with first-time moms admitted to the hospital is setting expectations as to what the hospital is like and what would be normal for their particular situation. Most moms don't understand how the hospital is set up and organized. Sharing the truths of hospital life will dispel the fear of the unknown. If you know what to expect next, you can cope with your labor and overall hospital experience in more manageable increments. I will help you learn about the sequence of care that is true for every patient in the hospital so you will have a compass as you move through the stages of care of your hospital birth.

Ultimately, the best way to prepare for a hospital birth is to prepare in three rhythms: mind, nurse, and spirit. Preparing the mind is the part about addressing expectations and knowing what to expect, realistically. Preparing for the nurse rhythm is simply to understand the value of your greatest resource during your hospital stay, your nurse. And the most transforming of your entire hospital experience will be preparing in your spirit. This book has been born out of a passion for the truth of these three rhythms, their power over how you perceive your hospital birth experience, and how you see yourself in your own story.

THE TRUTH ABOUT EXPECTATIONS

If you are a first-time mom getting ready to have a hospital birth, where would you get your idea of what to expect? Where do you look? Whose ideas influence you? What are you hoping will happen? I don't know about your experience, but there were plenty of people who were willing to share their birthing stories with me when I was pregnant. Most of the time, we get our expectations from listening to others. This can be on the TV or internet too.

There is no shortage of internet birthing advice out there, and it may be overwhelming to someone trying to sift out what is true when they have never experienced it before. The google searches for good birthing advice are so saturated with extreme opinions, promises of empowerment, fear tactics, and biases that it is almost impossible for the untrained eye to determine what is real truth.

Oftentimes, we listen to our families. Our mothers, sisters, cousins, and friends who have gone before us into the birth environment help shape our ideas as to what it is really like. Whether we mean it to or not, we are influenced by those close to us. Expectations can also come from physicians, birthing class educators, books, blogs, and

Pinterest. I hear patients tell me their expectations with statements like these:

> "My mom didn't get an epidural, so I probably won't either."
>
> "Women have been birthing babies for thousands of years; my body knows what to do."
>
> "I have a high pain tolerance; I shouldn't really need interventions."
>
> "I'm getting an epidural right away. I don't want to feel a thing."
>
> "I don't want a C-section, no matter what."

As a nurse, I am hearing the expectations coming through these sentences. They are not the same. They are different. But each woman speaking is communicating what they are expecting. What I have seen in postpartum is that the degree of their expectations matching their delivery seems to be associated with how they view their experience. Said another way, if a birth goes how the woman expected it to go, she will report a better birth experience. If a woman's experience does not meet her expectations, she is more likely to report a more negative view of her experience. This is just my postpartum observations, not a formal study, but from what I can tell, unmet expectations equal a more negative birth perception.

A patient's expectations are deeply tied to their sense of a positive outcome. That is subjective, and what defines a positive outcome can be different for every person. The woman who says, "I don't want a C-section, no matter what," is going to have a difficult time viewing her birth as positive in postpartum if she had to have a C-section. Similarly, the patient who didn't want to feel ANY pain at all, may say her epidural didn't work because she still felt the baby come out. Well, yes, a human being is still coming between your bladder and your rectum. An epidural can only mask so much, and normally with an epidural, one will feel the baby come out!

See what I mean though? Each expectation is different and very powerful in how we view our birth. Let me add another. The hospital has expectations too. The doctors and nurses define "a positive outcome" very differently than a patient will sometimes. "In health care, a positive outcome is the remediation of functional limitations or disability; the prevention of illness or injury; or an improvement in patient satisfaction."[1]

Our view of a positive outcome is having a healthy mom and a healthy baby. We embrace any set of interventions or changes that come in the labor experience to determine the best chance for everyone to be healthy through the process. It is inconsequential to us what route accomplishes this "positive outcome," although the same intervention might mean a "negative view" for the patient reviewing her own situation.

I have even seen medical care that has saved the lives of either mother or baby and STILL will hear the patient describe her hospital experience as poor. I believe that is because their expectation was tied to their wishes on their birth plan, and when the plans had to change, it was viewed as a failure of some kind.

A NURSE'S TAKE ON EXPECTATIONS

The prenatal education we are doing currently is not closing the gap between patient expectation and realistic nursing care. Most prenatal education deals with the biological process of birth and pain control strategies. Sometimes nurses aren't even the ones educating patients prenatally about hospital expectations. Patients are left to navigate the internet world and go to family/friends for help navigating birth. The problem is sometimes what the patient is expecting can be inconsistent with their specific situation.

For example, let's take our previously mentioned high-blood-pressure (hypertensive) patient from earlier. All of those labs and vitals might show a need for more intervention for the safety of mother and baby. Some ladies who have extreme blood pressures that do not immediately respond to treatment might end up on an IV medication called magnesium sulfate. This is a higher risk labor in which the treatment plan is intended to thwart medical complications such as seizure. It is not extremely common, but any provider in this discipline knows it is possible and will take action to prevent this complication, regardless of how far it strays from your birth plan.

This patient will indeed benefit from an earlier epidural because pain of contractions will contribute to higher blood pressures. So instead of birth balls and intermittent monitoring, this patient is going to have a different set of priorities for their care. Since high blood pressure can come on suddenly in the pregnant population, a patient really may have planned a different natural birth but now will need to revise expectations due to safety.

Also, high blood pressure doesn't seem to know when your baby shower is scheduled and has an uncanny ability to show up at inconvenient times for a hospital admission. It can be the definition of what you weren't expecting and truly had no control over, but yet it will require you to cope with a new reality.

Conversely, the healthy laboring mother who also has an IV might have her IV capped off and not attached to fluids, which will allow freedom of movement, showers, birth balls, and intermittent monitoring. Both patients have an IV, which is standard hospital protocol for a laboring mother, but their labors will look very different within that framework. Educating on expectations should be twofold when it comes to hospital deliveries. First, it is always helpful to understand the hospital setting and to know what is true for every single patient, regardless of the situation. Then, with a better understanding of the hospital in general, one should have expectations that match their specific situations.

I'm not a gambler. But I can imagine if I sat down at a card gaming table and kept betting on the hand I *wanted* vs. *the hand I am actually holding,* it would yield disastrous results. The same is true in labor. Your situation is the hand you've been dealt. To continue to try to bet on a birth plan that no longer fits your situation can be disastrous also. Expectations and plans should be tailored to the hand you are holding. In labor, that's your present condition when admitted to the hospital, not what you wish it would be.

ENTER THE NURSE

The start of me wanting to write this book was born out of the desire to have every patient talk to a labor nurse before their hospital delivery. Patients don't realize the gem who is assigned to them during every part of their stay in the hospital. I remember in nursing school one of my professors saying, "People are in the hospital because they need nursing care. Otherwise, they would be discharged to home."

Truthfully, you can look at every floor of the hospital and see this to be true. In the ER, we need nurses to be assigned to patients, to prioritize patient care, and to triage patients well. In medical/surgical floors of the hospital, the nurses are assigned to be at the bedside, using their training to specifically watch the flu patient or the patient fresh out of surgery so that no complications are missed. It is the vigilant eye of the nurse that will catch changes in conditions of each patient and will be instrumental with early intervention. In the ICU, there's a different level of specialty.

Respiratory therapists and medical doctors come in and out, but the nurse is the one continuously at the bedside monitoring complicated processes and medicinal interventions for the care of the patient. They know that patient so well, they are able to pick up on the slightest changes from the patient's baseline and save lives in doing so. I could go on and on. But the point is, when you have a trained eye at your bedside, you have a life-giving resource right at your fingertips. And sadly, usually, people who are patients do not understand the role of the nurse.

Preparing for birth in the rhythm of "your nurse" is learning about something you have probably never read on the internet or heard in any birthing education class. Understanding the role of your bedside labor nurse and appreciating her value is well spent time and preparation. I have tried to share with you in this book some ways to get to know her better and how she can help you through your labor experience.

Most of us are in this field of nursing because we have a heart not only for the medical, but for the humanistic care and touch of a bedside provider. We actually care about how you are feeling and want to address your fears. We want to serve your needs physically as well as emotionally and mentally. Your nurse most likely wants to actually bond with you and help make your labor experience all you are hoping it can be.

There's something else your nurse knows very well—the hospital environment. If you are new to the hospital, this is the person you want to ask your questions to. They can tell you so much about hospital function that it will serve you greatly if you learn to ask your nurse to help you set your expectations. They know not only the hospital well but also labor. They know not only labor well but so much about so many different types of patients and diagnoses and the individual importance of caring for each person differently.

They know how to take care of all types of patients, not only healthy ones. They are perfectly suited to explain your labor situation to you. They are the poker players who can explain to you your hand and help you play it the best way possible. They can explain in detail to you how your specific situation will be treated, what to expect, and how to move forward in it. Not only that, but they will be the one listening to you, how you respond to your personal situation, and can meet your needs emotionally as well as physically during your most intense moments. The nurse rhythm is so important because it can make your entire labor experience. Please believe me.

THE RHYTHM OF YOUR SPIRIT

If I wrote a book about hospital expectations (mind rhythm) and valuing your nurse (nurse rhythm) in your labor experience, you could definitely have a better hospital experience. No question there. But what makes the three-dimensional aspect of this book is the rhythm of your spirit. Aside from the wish that every patient could talk to a labor nurse before coming to the hospital, it is this spiritual aspect and the truths that became apparent to me that got me off my duff to write this book.

It all started with a small little book called, *A Shepherd Looks at Psalm 23*. For those of you who don't know, this psalm is written to highlight Jesus as the good shepherd who guards His flock of sheep (His people). Even through a quick read, you can see in the psalm how the shepherd is appreciated in providing for the sheep. It is a picture, a metaphor of sorts. The psalm uses a common phenomenon in those days, shepherding, to show a picture of something spiritual. But the author of this small book writes to explain the psalm differently and with amazing detail. The author is actually a shepherd. He does that job day in and day out. He is an expert at the physical job of shepherding.

His contribution to understanding the text is as a shepherd; he knows the behavior patterns of sheep. The author is detailed in explaining the patterns of sheep and how important it is to comprehend the sheep in order to understand the value of the shepherd's presence. It is understanding the sheep that provides this amazing ability to see yourself as the sheep in this analogy. Seeing yourself as the sheep postures you to appreciate the good shepherd with crystal clarity! It is truly my favorite book. So simple, yet so profound.

That got me thinking. Is God still in the business of teaching His people through everyday life? In the Bible, there are examples of metaphors like fishing for the fishermen, shepherd illustrations for those who knew sheep, illustrations of planting/harvesting for the agrarian mindset, and other parables taken out of everyday life for those who were listening. But in studying my job, what I have found is that the same concepts that can make us have better birthing experiences can in themselves be a physical picture of something spiritual. In fact, in looking at the truths of labor and delivery, I can see an amazing metaphorical analogy.

Just like the shepherd writing so his reader can understand the sheep, I find myself writing so you can better understand hospital birth. I can help you think of things that might be new to you and can help you truly have a better hospital birth experience. But I don't want to just teach you about sheep. I don't want you to just have a better birth. I want to share with you the spiritual truths that the physical act of birth illustrates so perfectly. I want to help you see and trust the Great Physician standing like a gentleman at your spiritual bedside.

Life is full of everyday "labors," and the same principles that will help you with physical labor and birth can prove to be life changing when applied to your life as a whole. This book is the sequence of how I've learned spiritual truths through a focused lens on the physical act of birth.

In this book, you will learn five core principles:

1. Your birth story is a series of unknowns that will unfold one piece at a time from beginning to end, and much which will be out of your control.

2. You will be assigned a guide to help you through birth at the hospital.

3. There will be an element of pain.

4. Your spirit will play heavily as to whether you view your birth story as positive or negative.

5. There is a spiritual thread that runs through the process of labor and birth, and the physical act of birth will highlight biblical truth concepts for better understanding.

I am privileged to be on this journey with you and am excited to prepare you for your transition to motherhood. It's an amazing rite of passage that needn't be marred with confusion or fear. I will help you prepare in a way different from your mother's Lamaze class. You will come to the hospital with a clearer understanding of its function, leaning on your nurse to be all she was meant to be for you, and if you're open to it, you just might be changed spiritually in the process.

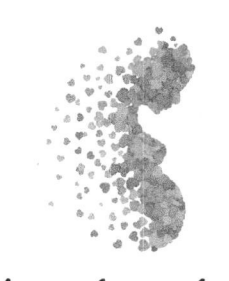

chapter two
HOSPITAL ORIENTATION: REALISTIC EXPECTATIONS ABOUT OUR BIRTH SETTING

THE STORK TOUR YOU REALLY NEED

The "stork tour" was hospital language for the large group of pregnant women and their partners walking around the Labor and Delivery unit to see where they will give birth. It has changed since the pandemic, but there used to be a weekly group of bright-eyed new moms who were given a tour of our labor unit. They were shown where they will register when they come to the hospital, where their triage room would be, what a labor room looked like, and where they would bond with their baby in postpartum. They basically got a geographical orientation.

A guide (in most cases, *not* a labor nurse) would give them a visual of what will be their birthing environment. In addition to learning where they could get ice, water, and snacks, at the end, the guide would gather them at the nursing station. As we were charting or watching fetal monitoring strips, these ladies would be given an opportunity to ask the nurses questions.

There usually would be an awkward moment of silence before someone would have the nerve to ask a question. They would all look around, daring each other with their eyes to ask the first question. But eventually there would be some questions.

> *"Can I bring my birth ball?"*
>
> *"Do we bring the car seat to the hospital?"*
>
> *"How does it work?"*
>
> *"Do you nurses call my doctor when I come in?"*
>
> *"Can I have a doula?"*
>
> *"Does everyone get epidurals here?"*
>
> *"Do I have to have an IV?"*

Weeks later, they would come in to get examined in triage and the questions would start again.

> *"Do I get my epidural now?"*
>
> *"How long is this going to take?"*
>
> *"Will the pain get worse than this?"*
>
> *"Can I take these monitors off?"*
>
> *"I have to get to a ten, right?"*

It is clear. Learning "where" the magic happens is good, but not good enough. Expectant moms should get a hospital orientation to the labor unit. Let me explain. *Orientation* is a word we use at the hospital, especially in the nursing profession. When I started as a new graduate nurse in the labor unit, I received an extensive orientation. I was assigned a preceptor who was to work with me continually for months as I learned to be a registered nurse in the discipline of labor and delivery. Yes, on the first day, I did learn where the locker room was, where to get food at the cafeteria, and how to sign on the computer system. But how unfair it would have been if my preceptor told me on my first day, "Okay, ask me all your questions."

The point is I needed to learn more about the job, the culture of the unit, where to find policies and procedures, and to have more experience with birth itself to even know what questions to ask. When you are learning something new in a new environment, it takes time to even know what it is you need to know more about! Now, an experienced labor nurse will get a three-day orientation to a new labor unit because they already know the job, they just need to know where to find things to *do* the job. They just need an orientation to the geography and maybe the culture and function of the unit.

For example, some hospitals have doctors on the unit twenty-four hours a day; at other hospitals, the doctor may be at home and the nurse has to call with enough time to get the physician to the birth of the baby. Different facilities have different policies/procedures, and an experienced nurse would need to know where to find those on a new job assignment.

To be successful, a nurse would need to know certain things about the unit that apply to every patient. Expecting moms are navigating the internet trying to be prepared for their birth. In the United States, 98.4 percent of women are having hospital births.[1] Yet, when I am at work laboring pregnant mothers, it seems the same percentage of women are unfamiliar with the flow of a hospital and how it works.

THE *heart* OF A BIRTH PLAN

I think most patients out there are spending time learning about the physiology of birth or pain control options. Some are trying to learn every nuance about labor and delivery and reading about things that don't even match their pregnancy situation.

You don't need a nursing degree or a six-month internship to prepare for your hospital birth. *You do need to know truths about the hospital that are true for every single patient.* The rest, you just need to know where to find the answer once you get there. Knowing the natural flow of the hospital unit and the team members working there will help you to squelch fear of the unknown. It also will help you to have the necessary information about your birthing setting, leading you to clearer questions.

LEARNING THE HOSPITAL SEQUENCE OF CARE—THE FLOW OF A LABOR UNIT

Hospital obstetrics has a very predictable sequence of care. How we care for a patient will follow a certain sequence, and it is true for everyone. Knowing this sequence, or hospital flow, will help you navigate where you are with the process of birth and what you can expect moving forward. I wanted to spend some time discussing the process because if you are not familiar with the inner workings of a hospital, it can help greatly with setting accurate expectations.

THE SEQUENCE OF CARE

Triage

This is the obstetrical ER. Any and everything related to pregnancy, usually a twenty-week gestation and beyond, goes first to obstetrical triage. This can go by different names depending on the hospital, but here are a few: labor and delivery triage, OB ED, or birthing center triage. Patients coming from home who want to be checked out at a hospital will first get an ID band at registration and go straight to triage. Doctors can also send patients to triage from regular doctor's appointments. Triage is the place where you will meet your first nurse. Your nurse will perform an assessment on you and assess the baby on the monitor. The purpose of triage is to determine whether you have a medical condition that warrants an admission to the hospital.

The nurse will form an impression and report findings to a physician. Depending on the setup at your hospital, you may see a doctor at your bedside discussing the plan, either to send you home or admit you to the hospital. Some hospitals may only have a triage nurse who communicates with the doctor via phone, and others may have a doctor available for triage consults day or night. There are many reasons why a pregnant mother may be admitted to the hospital, but active labor is the most obvious.

Admission

If you are admitted, you will be escorted to another room. You will meet another nurse. This will be your labor nurse. She will perform an admission assessment on you and ask you more computer questions than your initial triage questions. Your nurse will have you sign consents for treatment for the baby and start your IV. She will orient you to your new room and hopefully set expectations. Lots of questions are always asked about IVs. *Every patient who is admitted to the labor and delivery unit will get an IV.*

We use IV access for many reasons during labor. We use it to infuse fluids, give medicines, support the fetus during interruptions in oxygenation during labor, and to prepare for emergencies. Your IV can have fluids continuously running or it can be capped off. It is always better to allow IV access because it allows for staff to assist you rapidly during an emergency instead of being behind and trying to get an IV line when every minute may count.

Labor

Your labor will include everything happening from the time you are admitted to the hospital to the time you deliver your baby into the world. This can be a very short process if you are admitted in advanced labor, or it can be days long if you are a labor induction of any sort. This time period will include early labor, active labor, and the pushing phase (second-stage labor). Throughout this labor process, you will be taken care of by your labor nurse, perhaps many shifts of labor nurses. It is here, not during triage, where all epidurals take place.

A NOTE ON PAIN CONTROL

Once you are admitted to the labor unit as an "inpatient," you will have the option of two main medicinal modes of pain control.

1. Usually every labor unit will offer a short-acting narcotic IV pain control option. At our hospital, fentanyl is the drug of choice. For any IV pain medication, your nurse will review your baby on the monitor and make sure it is safe to give. This type of pain control works best for helping you to relax through contractions, but it will not take away all the

Hospital Orientation: Realistic Expectations about Our Birth Setting

pain of your contractions. The other limitation to this pain control is we usually do not give it if we feel the baby will deliver soon after the dose is given. Each dose will work for about an hour, but the more you have it, the less it will work for you. If you know you want a medicated labor, this option will work well to get you to the epidural placement.

2. The epidural is a procedure. Most patients do not realize this. I tell my patients from the time you tell us you want an epidural to the time you are pain-free can truly be thirty minutes to an hour or more. Preparation needed for an epidural is an IV that is working well to receive IV fluids to support your blood pressure during the procedure. Most anesthesiologists will want to see results of your blood work, looking specifically for platelets (clotting factors). These labs are part of the admission process and will be drawn when your nurse starts your IV initially. Once the anesthesiologist comes to the room, the procedure will start. Your nurse will support you through the whole thing.

3. She will help you position yourself so that placing the epidural is easier. Your epidural will be placed with a needle, but much like your IV placement, the needle is removed and there remains a tiny catheter in your back to deliver your medication. The needle does not stay in your back, and yes, you get numbing medicine. Some hospitals even give a patient-controlled button so you can dose yourself if you need more medicine. The epidural itself takes about fifteen to thirty minutes to place and feel some relief.

The idea of a good epidural block is to have some movement of your legs and great pain control. Some blocks are dense and the patient is very numb; others are lighter and the patient has great movement but may need their epidural topped off every now and then for great relief. The epidural will usually work well for the duration of your labor. Most patients with epidurals feel a great pressure or a sensation of needing to have a bowel movement as the baby descends. Patients will only feel this pressure at the end. Patients wanting a pain-free experience struggle with this and are frustrated when they realize the epidural didn't take away every sensation of having a baby. Plan on pressure close to delivery. It's a good sign.

You will have a urinary catheter placed to keep your bladder empty so the baby can descend. But don't worry, your epidural will be working before we place that, so no stress! Your nurse will take out the urinary catheter when it's time to push. We stop the epidural medicine after delivery of the baby and after any repairs are complete. It will take around two hours for you to be able to support your weight once the medicine is turned off, so please don't try to get up without a nurse! And that's the down and dirty for hospital medicine options.

Delivery

Vaginal: When your nurse feels that delivery is imminent, she will call for the doctor to attend your delivery. She will also call for a nursery nurse or team for the baby, and a technician might also come to your room to assist with instrumentation and patient care. You will meet your baby and finally get to see that precious life you took care of for so many months in utero! Most places are striving to become more mother/baby friendly and encourage skin-to-skin care and prioritize bonding during the first hour after birth. Some even do delayed cord clamping and delay routine baby care (like weights/measurements/medications/baths) so Mom and baby can bond and breastfeed.

Cesarean: This will be your time in the operating room. All of the same people will be present, except you will have three doctors: two obstetrical surgeons and one anesthesiologist. There will be your nurse and the NICU team along with the technician in the operating room as well. Depending on the situation, cesarean deliveries can vary tremendously from person to person. A controlled scheduled cesarean section is going to have a very calm relaxed routine feel to it. An emergent birth will seem chaotic because many team members need to be present to facilitate safe delivery on a time crunch.

Recovery

Recovery is roughly a two-hour period spent with your labor nurse recovering you from the delivery process. It is here where you will bond with your baby, and your nurse will watch your vitals and bleeding closely. You will recover both from a vaginal delivery or a cesarean section delivery. The hallmark of your recovery period not in the birth videos is something called uterine massage. Your nurse will need to massage your uterus often during your recovery period in order to prevent hemorrhage.

Firm uteruses bleed less, and when your nurse massages your uterus, it should firm up beneath her hand as she rubs on your belly near your belly button. She literally will rub your uterus every fifteen minutes for an hour after delivery, and it will continue throughout your postpartum stay, stretching out to every thirty minutes, hourly, every four hours, every eight hours, etc. Your nurse is looking at how much bleeding is visible and taking measurement of the top of your uterus, making sure bleeding isn't collecting inside. Each hospital has its own policy on this, but you should know to expect it and that it is good care. Truthfully, this is not pleasant and is not usually on the birthing videos but is a necessary part of your recovery time.

Postpartum

When you are stable and recovered from delivery, you will be transferred to a clean new room for postpartum. During delivery, especially for first-time mothers, there usually is some type of perineal tearing or lacerations. If they are repaired, the sutures will dissolve. But the first time you get up to go pee after having a baby is never on the birthing videos either. It is a vulnerable time your nurse will help you with, and she will show you how to soothe your perineum.

Postpartum is a time when you learn to breastfeed and care for your baby. You will have a nurse assigned to you during this time as well, but they will have many other patients. It is best that you pick a support person to stay the night with you who will help you with baby care. You will start the process of self-care and develop a routine with your baby you can feel comfortable with at home.

There are many tasks in postpartum care that must be completed with the baby before discharge and will happen during this phase of care. Many of these hospital tasks before discharge will be from different people in different departments and will not be coordinated. Examples of people who will visit you before your discharge while in postpartum: pediatricians, dietary, lab, nurses, obstetricians, lactation consultants, birth certificate clerk, photographer, newborn hearing screen specialist, and social services if warranted. It will feel like a revolving door before discharge. When I was a nurse on night shift, I told my patients that between the hours of 1:00 a.m. and 5:00 a.m. were hours of protected sleep. Please try to sleep during that time because the revolving door starts around 5:00 a.m.

Discharge

This is the end of your hospital stay. A nurse will go over all the education for your journey home, and you will receive follow-up appointments. You are on your way home!

This is a basic overview of the process as a whole. Many patients have questions about this process when they get to the hospital, so I wanted to start sharing the inner workings with you so you can know what to expect. Of course, these steps are fluid. Obviously, if you come into the hospital 9 cm dilated and ready to have a baby, we are going to get ready for your little one. I assure you, though, your nurse is still going to have to perform steps from the triage and admission. It just will be condensed and quick. So, all the steps are valid for each patient, although it may look different for varying scenarios.

Understanding the Professionals in This Setting

As a labor nurse, I see so many patients asking the same question: "When does the doctor come in?" It is a surprise to many patients that the doctor isn't at the bedside laboring with them or that their role doesn't include more time at the bedside. I wanted to write this overview of the hospital staff on a labor and delivery unit to help you mentally set realistic expectations for your hospital birth. Here is a brief description of the people you may encounter during your time in the hospital to have your baby.

The Team

OB/GYN Physicians—These are medically trained doctors who specialize in women's health and obstetrics (care of women giving birth). It will vary at different institutions, but the main idea of how doctors function in the hospital setting on the labor unit is the same. *There is one doctor responsible for many patients.* In one type of setup, there is a doctor working an assigned shift, and during that shift, they will be responsible for all laboring patients on the unit (postpartum as well).

There is another type of setup where a doctor is responsible for his own patients in the clinic (your regular pregnancy appointments) as well as in the hospital and will share "call" with other doctors as part of a group during the nights and evenings. Doctors physically can't be ready for action 24 hrs/day, 7 days/week. But since babies come 24 hrs/day, 7 days/week, they will do some type of patient sharing with other physicians. There is a high likelihood that you will not have the same physician for your delivery as you do for your prenatal care. This is often a surprise to patients.

Certified Nurse Midwives—This is a graduate-level trained nurse who specializes in birth. These are practitioners who help attend deliveries and can function in the place of a doctor for a healthy population of patients. They function with and report to the MD responsible for the patients. Not all facilities will have them, and there are other midwifery designations that exist with different qualifications outside of a hospital setting.

Labor Nurses—This is a registered nurse who has specialized in labor and delivery. This is the person who is dedicated and assigned to be at your bedside for most of your care experience. Each nurse will have one or two labor patients depending on the stage of labor. During your labor, your nurse will most likely have two patients to look after. Once you start the pushing phase, your nurse will be all yours. She will be with you continuously throughout pushing, during the delivery of your baby, and usually your recovery period as well. *Ninety-nine percent of your hospital experience will be with your labor nurse.* Your labor nurse will know you better than anyone else on the staff because she will easily spend the most time with you.

It is your labor nurse who will form relationships with you. It is your labor nurse who will be answering most of your questions, hearing your concerns, performing your hands-on care, helping you with positioning, pain control, and a whole host of other things that never make the birth videos. By spending the most time with you, your labor nurse knows you so well that she is able to function as your advocate. She can speak to what is good for you as your labor unfolds. Knowing one or two patients so well is valuable because she will be reporting to the attending physician who has many patients to whom he/she is responsible.

The plan of care will be communicated between the doctor and nurse, and the nurse becomes the eyes and ears of the physician who is not at the bedside. It is the nurse's expertise that is trusted to evaluate how a patient is progressing with the plan of care, identify any problems needing to be treated, and communicate the needs of the patient to the doctor. If a doctor has questions about a patient's progress, he/she talks to the nurse assigned to that patient.

I assure you, it is your nurse who will make your hospital experience by listening to you, speaking up for you, coordinating your care, having tough conversations with you, explaining care to you, and being present at your bedside with you. This personal effort can result in a relational connection that is very fulfilling for both the patient and the nurse. It will help you immensely as your labor in the hospital to value your bedside nurse. I feel so strongly about this that I dedicated the whole next chapter to it!

Here is a picture of the reporting structure in the hospital. You can see the doctor is responsible for many patients but removed from the hands-on care of the patient. It is very important that doctor/nurse trust is maintained to keep the standard of care at a high level. That means there is a level of expertise from your nurse that the doctors depend on and will affect your care.

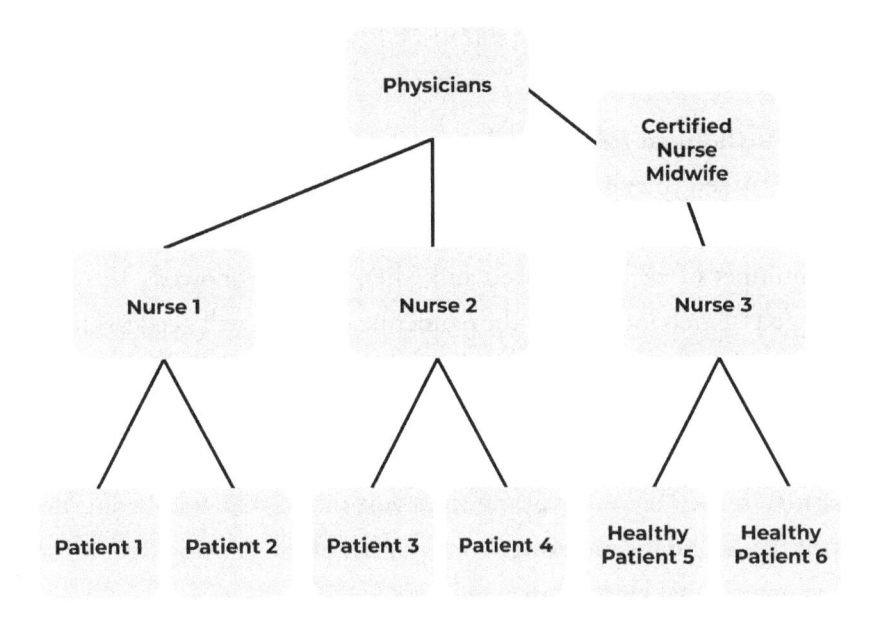

Hospital Orientation: Realistic Expectations about Our Birth Setting

```
                    Physicians
                   /    |    \
                  /     |     Certified Nurse Midwife
                 /      |              \
             Nurse 1  Nurse 2         Nurse 3
             /  \      /  \           /   \
        Pt 1  Pt 2  Pt 3  Pt 4   Healthy   Healthy
                                 Patient 5  Patient 6
```

HOSPITAL RULES

Each of these professionals have education and licenses that correspond with their scope of practice. Each professional has governing bodies they answer to for their choices during your care experience. There are standards of care that define competence each professional must adhere to as they care for you. A professional will tell you what you *need* to hear, not what you may *want* to hear as your labor unfolds. A hard truth is better than a sweet lie, and they will not lie to you if they see something is unsafe.

If they feel your situation is requiring a change in care in order to stay within the realm of reasonable competence, to guide you to a healthy mom and healthy baby, they will make that change. They will choose safety always, not just for your safety, but because they will protect their license as well. Unfortunately, labor and delivery is a medical discipline with high risk for lawsuit because everyone expects a perfect birth.

There are hospital rules as well that may be different from facility to facility. When you are having a hospital birth, you need to understand there will be rules for you as well. For example, we have rules about the number of visitors allowed and when they are allowed. This has changed tremendously with the pandemic, and you will need to know the specific rules for your birth hospital about COVID restrictions, visitors, mask wearing, and COVID testing. Most hospitals will accommodate many birth plan's wish lists such as music, birth balls, mirrors, scents, etc. One of the rules you should know up front: no open flames. So if candles were on your list of the relaxing, you must plan on artificial battery-operated ones.

THE ELECTRONIC FETAL MONITOR

Truthfully, this electronic fetal monitor is the subject of much heated debate amongst natural birthers vs. hospital birthers. I have a special certification in electronic fetal monitoring and wanted to share some truths with you regarding it. Truth: your hospital birth will involve electronic fetal monitoring. Your situation, where you are in the labor process, and the results of your monitoring will determine how much monitoring you will experience. If you are a young healthy mother without any complications and in latent labor (beginning of the labor process), you might experience less monitoring.

If you are experiencing regular contractions and cervical dilation as time progresses, you are in active labor and will have a continuous electronic fetal monitoring experience. If you are a person with any medical conditions with your pregnancy (diabetes, hypertension, low amniotic fluid, twins, preterm labor, etc.) or an induction of labor, you will experience continuous monitoring. Continuous meaning it's always there.

The monitoring has changed over the years as far as technology. Some facilities now have cordless monitoring or remote monitoring allowing more movement/freedom during labor. But as with any technology, all come to have limitations and none are perfect. The most common setup is the two monitors strapped to your belly, one for ultrasound to trace the fetal heart rate and the other to monitor when the contractions are occurring and how long they are lasting. The monitor determines the fetal heart rate and traces it over time on a printed paper (we also have it electronically).

The monitor tracing over time reveals a pattern that we have come to interpret. In fact, we actually have interpretive language for your tracing we are responsible for knowing and interpreting correctly. The National Institute of Child Health and Human Development standardized the language for how every professional in the discipline of labor and delivery reads and communicates about your fetal heart rate strip.[2]

We are responsible for this language, and as a patient, you probably will hear the doctors and nurses speaking this foreign language at your bedside. That is a good thing, but most patients are caught off guard when these terms are spoken at the bedside. I want you to know to expect it. Even though you may not understand this foreign language, your nurse can explain your strip to you as needed.

Believe it or not, the tracing can tell us about the interplay between the sympathetic and parasympathetic nervous system. By studying the tracing, professionals can tell if the baby is giving reassuring signs of adequate oxygenation, thus ruling out concerning problems. It also can tell us if the baby is experiencing interruptions in oxygenation during your labor that require intervention. The important thing to understand is the electronic monitor *rules out* possible complications quite well.

If you know the language of the fetal monitor and can interpret the fetal heart rate tracing properly, identifying a fetal strip that is without problem is relatively easy. Conversely, a fetal strip with undeniable dangerous problems is also easy to spot by professionals. What is important for you to know as a patient is that a majority of all labor fetal heart rate strips will fall in a large "middle" category. Most patients at some point in their labor will have oxygenation interruptions as part of the labor process.

Some will present themselves as a normal part of labor and will require no intervention. Others will require simple interventions such as changing the mother's position. Others will require a keener eye and judgment over time. This large middle patient population is where the expertise of the physician and nurse collaboration becomes evident. If a tracing is no longer giving those reassuring signs that the fetus is well-oxygenated, the professionals must evaluate how serious the tracing is and make the shortest plan toward delivery.

Once the monitor stops showing the reassuring signs, the doctor and nurse will course your path for delivery using their best judgment. It is true the monitor is great at predicting the absence of problems. It is not predictive, however, of ensuring a dangerous outcome is 100 percent present. That means as the provider is making judgments for delivery, there may be times when we are concerned about a tracing and the baby comes out fine. This is how monitoring can get a bad rap for increased the cesarean-section rate.

Hospital Orientation: Realistic Expectations about Our Birth Setting

Truthfully though, a doctor is going to decide for your welfare and the best intentions of your baby. The monitor is not perfect, but it is the best we have. Because it's the best we have and it's not perfect, it requires the skilled judgments of providers to do the best they can in their human frame to give you the birth plan of your dreams. They also will weigh the tracing with their education and governing bodies of authority and will make the safest decision protecting them in the court of law as well.

When I am at the bedside with my patients I tell them the fetal heart rate tracing has a basic language of interpretation amongst professionals. Some things we may ask you to do, like change your position, will be in response to your fetal heart rate tracing. That would be normal. So, when should you be concerned about your fetal heart rate tracing? I liken the experience to being on a plane. I am uncomfortable with turbulence. Just the slightest bit of it freaks me out totally. I try to watch the flight attendants. If I'm freaking out, but they are laughing and serving drinks, then I can take a cue that we are not in a death-defying free fall. However, if the flight attendants are strapped in and have an urgency about their faces, then I can interpret that we are in a situation out of the norm.

Labor is much like that. It is common for your nurse to respond to your tracing. It is also common for more than one nurse to respond because you are on central monitoring and all the nurses on the unit can see every patient's fetal heart rate strip. But if there are four nurses, a doctor, and someone is unplugging your bed cords, then most likely there is a situation in which we need to act quickly and save explanations for later. Your nurse is your flight attendant. Watch her. She doesn't have to teach you the entire fetal heart rate language to help you interpret your strip. She is also a wealth of information about your fetal heart rate strip and can help you know what to expect as your labor story unfolds on and off the monitor.

THE HOSPITAL ILLUSION OF CONTROL

A simple search of the definition of control on dictionary.com will reveal this definition: "Con·trolled, con·trol·ling—to exercise restraint or direction over; dominate; command: to hold in check; curb."[3] The idea of "control" is HUGE in the birth room. So I ask you: Who is in control of your birth experience? Is it you? There are a lot of websites out there promising patient empowerment and showing you how to "take control" of your birthing experience. They make me nervous.

Educating a patient on defense strategies to manipulate your hospital circumstances to your advantage and trying to control hospital staff in myriads of ways will not help you have a fulfilling hospital birth experience. The problem with these strategies is they often will set up hospital staff as the enemy. If you are having a hospital birth, you will not have a positive birthing experience if you believe the doctors and nurses are intending to harm you. You can take that one to the bank.

If the hospital staff is the enemy, then you are planning for a scared patient, in pain, to also be responsible for defending herself against unwanted harm during the most vulnerable, painful time in her life. At a time when you are at most uncomfortable in a new environment, in pain physically, and emotionally vulnerable, no one should ask you to be at your best with a militant defensive strategy.

This is how women end up feeling like failures in postpartum because they "weren't strong enough" during their labor and they feel like they "failed" because they had an intervention they weren't planning on. The amount of postpartum false guilt is ridiculous when birthing with these strategies, and it is completely unfair. It is unfair to assign guilt/blame to a mother because she listened to the hospital staff and had an intervention she truly needed, mostly because of circumstances that were out of her control to begin with.

I guess it takes one to know one here. When I had my first son, I was not yet a nurse. I had taken a birthing preparation class that viewed labor as an athletic event. It was proposed that if you followed the prescribed suggestions, planned and prepared physically for your birth, and learned what hospital interventions to refuse, then you could have an unmedicated natural birth. I was hooked because at that time in my life, before pregnancy, I was in the gym two hours a day and really felt I had a great chance of being disciplined enough to "prepare" for birth physically.

I followed said plan religiously. I recorded all my nutrition, exercised, and read everything I could get my hands on about natural birth. I really felt I was ready, even when people I knew made fun of my plan. I just knew I was going to be all right. *I mean really…people have been doing this for thousands of years*, I thought. Plus, I had been praying about my plan for months and felt confident my petitions would not go unnoticed.

I'll shorten my birth story for you. I went two weeks overdue. I took castor oil to beat my medical induction, possibly more than I should have. I had the worst diarrhea of my life. In driving to my hospital of choice that had the midwives, the bridge I needed to cross was closed for road work at 2:00 a.m. I found myself on the floor of a local firehouse literally on a white sheet with blood running down my arm as a perceived newbie started my IV. I was there because my husband listened to the screaming pregnant lady on her knees from the floor of our Ford F150. Yes, that was me, and I was still trying to strategize this thing!

I rationalized that they would let an ambulance through the closed bridge. So naturally, I needed to get to an ambulance. I was hoping that was true as I asked my husband to take me to a firehouse. Firehouse => Ambulance => Getting over the bridge => Hospital with my midwives => Natural unmedicated delivery. See? There was still a chance!

While trying not to soil myself while on hands/knees on the floor of the firehouse with terrible back labor, I heard the voice of a guy I went to high school with who happened to be working that night. I think I remember him saying, "Maria, is that you?"

I took a humiliating ambulance ride I will never fully disclose in writing. When I got to the hospital, I was 3 cm dilated, and whoever checked me told me my baby was in a bad position. Then, my first perceived failure: I got an epidural.

Twenty some odd hours later, with every intervention known to man, I pushed for over three hours and after a doctor came in to talk to me about "other ways of having this baby," I delivered. What I didn't understand was my baby's strip must have looked awful, hence the million interventions and the crowd of professionals in my room. My baby was born struggling and had meconium aspiration and was in the NICU for eight days. In postpartum, I was using my nursing pillow not for nursing, but for sitting on since I found out later I fractured my coccyx during delivery.

I was left to pick up the pieces of my shattered expectations and rationalize what on earth went wrong. Not being a nurse then, and not being able to sift out what was mine to control and what was completely out of my control, I started blaming myself. I blamed myself for not being strong enough to handle birth. I felt ashamed and embarrassed since I had told everyone I wanted a natural unmedicated birth. I thought the things I had done could have hurt my baby, and the thoughts were haunting. And then there was this, "Lord, are You even there? And if You are, what was that?!"

Aside from this being a very entertaining story for my labor nurse friends at 3:00 a.m. on night shift, having this birth experience has made me acutely aware of connecting with my patients in postpartum. I do now what I wish a nurse had done for me when I was in bewilderment during my postpartum days. I pay special attention to the patients who come in with a strong birth plan idea, have circumstances out of their control, and are left to adapt to changing situations. I literally pull up a chair, hold their hand, look into their weepy eyes, and tell them to "release" themselves from that which they never had control over in the first place.

Birth is a wild adventure. You don't know all the events and nuances that will make up the details of your birth story. Your birth story will be a series of unfolding events as labor progresses that will be unknown to you, and it will challenge you to release yourself from that which you do not control.

EDUCATION DOES NOT EQUAL CONTROL

It is a common belief among labor nurses that the hardest patients to take care of are nurses and teachers. The reason is no matter how much formal education you have or how many books you read on birth, this premise is still true: Education does not equal control. In fact, the wrong prenatal education or the wrong application of birth information that does not fit your personal labor situation can be dangerous.

Education can betray you in that bed. I have seen it. In fact, I have seen labor nurses crying before their own cesarean because they have seen too much and know the possibilities of what can go wrong. In fact, it is their knowledge, not their situation, that breeds fear. "But surely the doctors are in control, right? I mean someone has got to be the captain around here!"

Thinking the doctor is in control is an illusion. Doctors or nurses do not have control over your labor because they wear white coats or scrubs and have accolades after their names. In fact, every medical provider in this discipline would tell you the only constant in labor and delivery is change. Some patients who you think will deliver fast, will plug along. Some who you think will have difficult labors, surprise you and go from 3 cm to complete and are pushing before you know it! Some patients who you didn't think were going to be that sick show very concerning lab results, and their plan of care needs to change. Some babies are bigger than we think. Some babies are smaller. Some babies are head down as expected, and some patients come in breech. Change!

Hospital language is we "manage" patients. In fact, a nurse will say, "Who's managing this patient?" meaning, who is the provider I'm getting a plan of care and orders from? Is it the midwife or the physician on call? We don't say, "Who's controlling this patient's labor?" Someone is responsible for "managing" the patients. Let me explain how this works.

You will come into the hospital labor unit with what we call a baseline, a place of beginning. This is the story that has unfolded during your prenatal care experience. All those lab tests, appointments, urine samples, and ultrasounds have put together pieces of your unfolding story. When you come in to triage to be evaluated for admission to labor, you will be assigned a provider (doctor or midwife). A triage nurse will gather information by hearing what brought you in today, taking new vitals, collecting a new urine sample, and watching your baby on the monitor.

It's with this information that she gives a report to the doctor. The doctor will evaluate your current situation coupled with your prenatal information and will form a plan of care. It is here that education becomes important. The providers will use their education, accolades, and experience to evaluate your entire "presenting" situation and preserve safety for you and your baby. The doctor has a duty to act on his/her education and is ultimately responsible for the decisions made on behalf of the patient.

"Managing" a patient is the act of receiving all the information about a labor over time as it unfolds and adjusting the plan of care accordingly. This discipline is fluid. Even after you are admitted and labor progresses, new information will come to light and may require a change in how it is "managed." Your nurse is trained to recognize the unfolding of new information, evaluate the change in your situation, and collaborate with the doctor if change in the management plan is indicated. The hospital labor culture is very flexible with change in this discipline. We are extremely comfortable with change.

We know we could be eating lunch and in thirty seconds flat can be running out to the parking lot to deliver a baby in someone's car. (Yes, it happens.) We are so comfortable with change that it is almost casual with us. A doctor can casually walk into a patient's room and make a simple statement that is completely casual to them: "Your baby's heart rate is showing that the baby is not tolerating labor. Because we are not close to delivery, I am recommending we do a cesarean section." And then he walks out, and the absolute wheels come off emotionally in that room. Here's why.

THE PROBLEM: LABOR WILL CHALLENGE YOUR PRECONCEIVED EXPECTATIONS

There's something in psychology called the normalcy bias. Normalcy bias is a psychological state of denial people enter in the event of a disaster, as a result of which they underestimate the possibility of the disaster actually happening and its effects on their life and property. Their denial is based on the assumption that if the disaster has not occurred until now, it will never occur. An estimated 70 percent of people are affected by normalcy bias. Of the remaining 30 percent, half the people freak out, while the remaining show presence of mind and do the right thing.[4] (You can read more about it here: "An Insight into the Concept of Normalcy Bias in Psychology.")

This article explains why in a hurricane or flood, people will not heed warnings and can suffer loss because they are in denial that it can be "that bad." They believe it will be "like any other hurricane" and plan to ride it out, even though there are severe warnings plenty of time in advance to evacuate and minimize loss. People know a bad outcome is possible; they just don't believe it will happen to them.

I believe there is a similar phenomenon in labor. This explains why people will intellectually understand there are true medical reasons for needing an operative birth, but they just don't think it will happen to them. Ladies *do* believe it when they hear there are women who had a cesarean because the baby wasn't tolerating labor. They also believe there are women who have high blood pressure, diabetes, cholestasis, placenta previa, abruption, postpartum hemorrhage, or other conditions requiring medical-style births with more intervention. They believe it exists; they just don't believe it will happen to them.

So, what we end up with is a patient who came into the hospital with certain expectations for perfection. She is giving birth in an environment unfamiliar to her, which creates anxiety. She is listening to medical speak, which sounds like a foreign language. She may feel like she has to protect herself from "intervention happy" hospital people to have a decent experience. And none of this is what she was expecting!

Medical people get a bad rap and are accused of ruining a perfectly good birthing experience with their suggestions of things like cesareans because most patients assume they would not be one of the people who need one. A casual mention of a cesarean by a doctor is a natural progression of the provider weighing the information as it unfolds over time as you are in the hospital. Labs can change, a patient's response to an induction method can change, and how the fetus appears on the monitor can change.

A physician is responsible for many patients at a time, all whose situations are fluid and changing. His/her job is to manage each patient in the safest way possible, because they have ultimate authority when it comes to the decision-making for that particular patient, and they are the most educated person to do it.

They are not going to be at your bedside holding your hand and necessarily caring about how you "feel" about the changes in your labor. They usually make decisions impersonally based on the factual information in front of them coupled with what they know to be risks moving forward, and they will choose the path of limited risks. The patient, however, who honestly may have expected the doctor to be bedside laboring her (meaning always at the bedside as some sort of emotional guide or support) is now in a crisis. It is becoming apparent that what she expected is not happening and may not even be possible. She is feeling out of control and truly never thought this would happen to her. To get to the heart of solving this dilemma, every patient should answer this question in advance of their labor. Read it slowly and think about it: *Who is in control?*

We already have established you are *not* in control of the circumstances that form your birth story. Remember the bridge that was closed for road work? I rest my case. We have also established that doctors being in control is an illusion. They don't know the circumstances that will unfold from beginning to end to be your birth story any more than you do. They are simply "managing" your labor as it changes and new information is obvious. So who IS in control? This is a spiritual question, not a physical question. It has become obvious to me over the years that the spiritual aspect of what one believes about themselves as a being will absolutely affect their perceived birth experience.

SPIRITUAL TRUTH—YOUR LABOR AND BIRTH STORY IS AN "ASSIGNMENT"

When I was a young mom of a two-year-old boy (yes, the same boy who broke my butt!), we learned my son had a new diagnosis of nephrotic syndrome, or kidney disease. I was not a nurse at that time and was overwhelmed with this new truth in our lives. Our lives completely changed overnight as this was discovered. I did not understand the diagnosis really and was completely frightened. My imagination had all kinds of ideas as to what this might mean and all kinds of questions I was actually afraid to ask, chief of them being, "Can he die?"

I am going to share with you my story from my source of truth. I am a Christian, and my source of truth is the Bible. At the time, I was a very new Christian and was just so new at my new relationship with God. I remember we had our pastor over to talk with my husband and me as we were trying to digest this new life. I don't remember every word of this conversation, but there was a truth nugget I learned that changed my life, literally. He said, "Being a parent of a sick child is an assignment."

An assignment. I thought and thought about what kind of assignment this could be. What does it mean? An assignment to me is something given to you, not something you choose. I understood I was to use everything I already knew about God and purpose it specifically for my "assignment." I had to go back and really study what I believed about God and why I believed it. Then I had to understand that "religion" had to become "relationship" in order for me to walk it out in my earthly "assignment." Let me explain.

So, I believed God is the Creator and is in control. That means I had to face that God was in control, even though my kid was sick. I believed God had specifically allowed this boy to be born to me. I was handpicked for raising a two-year-old with a kidney condition. I had to study about what being a Christian meant in relation to walking in this new given assignment. Using what I believed spiritually gave me a framework to work within when figuring out how to move through the day to day.

Faith in God to me became waking up every day, trusting God would be with me all day. It was not just church on Sunday and growth group on Wednesdays. It was my seeking Him on Monday as my two-year-old complained of back pain. It was praying on Tuesday that I would see His presence living out our "lab draws" for the day. It was reading His Word on Wednesday before driving to Children's Hospital for specialty care. After looking around the waiting room, I was thanking Him on Thursday that my son has a manageable kidney condition. It was praying for those other moms with special-needs children who I saw with much harder assignments.

I knew the Bible says He knows the beginning from the end and has promised to never leave me or forsake me.[5,6] Now, I needed these verses to jump off the pages and become true for me personally every day. I learned to walk forward in trust on a daily basis with my sick kid, never knowing what tomorrow was going to be like, just trusting to see God in "today." Truthfully, I didn't know how long my son would be sick. I thought he might be sick for the rest of his life. It was too hard to have the correct perspective looking at this large assignment: I might be the parent of a sick kid for the rest of his life. I learned to literally break it down day to day.

So, my prayers changed to this: "God would You please be with us today as we go to the lab to get his blood drawn? Would You just show us You are with us? Give us the perfect person to draw his blood today. Help me be all You would have me be as a mother to my son today." Then this would happen: the lab person would take my two-year-old and blow up a glove to make a balloon for him to hold and squeeze while he got his blood drawn. And my kid wouldn't cry. Or the next time, we had a girl who would have my two-year-old hold all the blood tubes, and he got to call out the color he wanted her to use next. And my kid wouldn't cry.

Now, some would say, "Okay, seriously, what a coincidence." But let me tell you, when you string day after day, week after week, year after year together, and you are trusting God for comfort as you walk through the unknown of your earthly assignment, you look for patterns.

I have stories of those years when I knew God to be walking with me in that assignment, teaching me to lean on Him and trust Him. Chief of which was my son entering remission from his kidney disease in 2009 without medical explanation. For whatever reason, that assignment ended for me, and believe me, we were so thankful. I didn't want my kid to be sick, of course, but having to rely on what I knew to be true spiritually to live out this earthly assignment, taught me to trust God.

I don't believe I would have understood it as clearly as I did when literally it was all I had. I didn't know that everything would be okay. But it taught me the truth in this: "Trust in the LORD with all your heart, and do not lean on your own understanding. In all your ways acknowledge Him and He will make straight your paths" (Proverbs 3:5–6).[7]

I started to see that we all have assignments. Some of us have illnesses like cancer. Some have disabilities. Some have circumstances that are temporary I see as "assignments" like lost jobs, financial hardships, marital problems, or child-rearing challenges. I have noted that in any of these arenas, whether they are financial hardships, relational challenges, or physical sufferings, the lessons are the same. It is an assignment to use what you truly believe about *who* is in control to walk through the day to day of a hardship.

OUR LABOR ASSIGNMENT

In later years, I would become a nurse and would carry this train of thought into my nursing shift. Let me tell you a truth about the hospital that is the epitome of irony. In the hospital, nurses get "assignments." Seriously, that's what we call it. We come in every day and go into the locker room and change into our scrubs. While we are changing and preparing for the shift, we have no idea what our assignment will be. We take all of our knowledge, training, education, and experience, and with our scrubs on, we go to a meeting called a "huddle" where we are given our assignments for the shift.

It sounds like this:

> *"Maria, your assignment is a primip (first-time mom) in room 105 who wants an epidural. She's getting prepared now and is 5-cm dilated."*
>
> *"Nurse #2, you have a lady in triage who is getting prepared for a cesarean section for breech presentation."*
>
> *"Nurse #3, you have a lady who delivered vaginally an hour ago. Please finish her recovery."*
>
> *"Nurse #4, you have three mom-and-baby couplets in postpartum, one who is trying to go home today."*

This truth became so profound to me. It was a physical illustration of a spiritual concept. Physically, we are going to use all of our knowledge and training and apply it to our assignments. Here's another fact:

we nurses know that as we put on scrubs in the locker room, we have no idea where the situation of our assignments will take us. We understand things could change at any moment as labor unfolds with our patient. Maybe I am assigned a labor patient who delivers quickly. Maybe I will go to the operating room with my patient. Maybe my patient has an uncomplicated, natural birth. Maybe my patient is an intense medical patient who needs special care. When I first get my assignment, I just don't know where my work shift will lead.

That is because each patient is also going to get a labor assignment. As a nurse, I am coming alongside a lady living out her own labor assignment. Our paths cross for a limited amount of time as I am trying to make a difference in my patient's story. Rarely do you control the circumstances of your labor. Over time, your labor unfolds into a birth story managed by physicians, supported by nurses, and walked through by the patients themselves. We all are actually walking out assignments given to us, none of us truly knowing where it will end up until the end of the story. It's actually a beautiful thing.

It is the same spiritually. When you have a situation you have no control over, it will challenge you to use *what you believe* to cope. I don't know what the circumstances were that led you to your pregnancy, but I know we all have a story. Maybe your pregnancy itself was unexpected and you are wrestling through what you believe and how to cope moving forward. Maybe your pregnancy was planned but you are anxious about labor. Maybe there are extenuating circumstances with your pregnancy that are unexpected and you are trying to shift your expectations about your delivery.

Wherever you see yourself, let me tell you an old truth that has been proven true at the bedside in more ways than I can count: For me,

THE *heart* OF A BIRTH PLAN

God is in control. He has been the God of the womb since Genesis, and without being distracted, we would do well to remember the beginning.

> For you formed my inward parts; you knitted me together in my mother's womb. I praise you, for I am fearfully and wonderfully made. Wonderful are your works; My soul knows it very well. My frame was not hidden from you, when I was being made in secret, intricately woven in the depths of the earth. Your eyes saw my unformed substance; in your book were written every one of them, the days that were formed for me, when as yet there was none of them. [8] | Psalm 139:13–16

You were absolutely chosen for this time and place, to be the mother of the baby inside you. Just as each eye, finger, leg, and toe are being formed on your baby, so will your pregnancy story be woven together. It will be a faith journey, and like any faith journey, you don't get to see the end until you get there. As you get closer to the delivery of your baby, I hope you can lean into the realities of hospital life. It is its own breed, but it can be beautiful. Your labor will be fashioned and formed by the circumstances surrounding it.

But to truly have a positive perception of your own birth story, you might want to answer the spiritual questions. Who is in control? In believing this, what does it mean for me to trust in this assignment of my labor and birth? Getting to the heart of a birth plan will mean answering the spiritual questions not talked about at your clinic visits. But walking through a physical assignment with spiritual confidence will make a huge difference in how you see yourself in your own birth story.

chapter three
AN ORIENTATION TO YOUR NURSE

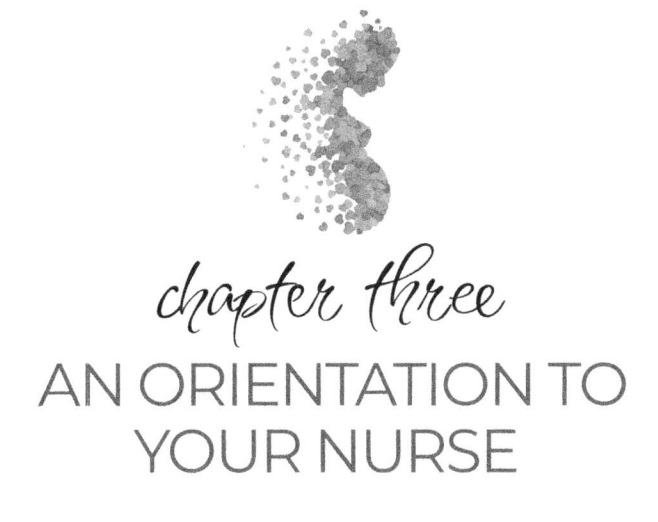

THE GUIDE

When I was preparing to write this book, I was listening to a podcast by Christy Wright. She had a guest speaker from Storybrand Marketing, Donald Miller, on the show that day. The guest was talking about the plot of any good movie having a person who has a problem. That person meets a guide who gives them a plan to solve their problem. The person is able to implement said plan and solves their problem, becoming the hero in their own story.[1]

It was so perfect for me to hear that day. I had been trying to describe what a nurse does in the hospital for a laboring patient. When I heard this, it was kismet in solving my own problem of communicating the value of a good nurse in labor and delivery. A good nurse in labor and delivery is literally your guide assigned to you to help you through birth. She is your guide to recognize problems if they come up and can give you a plan for solutions. She will tell you the truth and help to empower you to understand your given labor situation. She is there to help you, and believe me, you need her input into your situation. She is your Yoda and has wisdom to share at your bedside.

Sadly, in my opinion, the value of a good labor and delivery nurse goes unnoticed by most patients. Hospitals everywhere are trying to figure out how to have their patients perceive better hospital birthing experiences, and I believe they are overlooking the most pivotal asset to a patient's experience. It is the value of the nurse. They just don't know how to connect the patient's expectations *prehospital,* to the patient's experience *in* the hospital when it comes to the nurse. It is a missed opportunity to not be communicating with you before your labor experience how valuable your nurse can be for you during your hospital birth. I believe this chapter really may help to close the gap here and provide a much-needed orientation of what a labor nurse is and what she actually brings to your bedside.

> **Fact:** *99 percent of your hospital experience will be with your bedside nurse.* Most patients are surprised by this and are expecting something else. I'm not actually sure what they are expecting. Some people just think the nurse is there to give meds, fluff your pillow, and fill your water pitcher. Others have no idea what to think of their nurse's role in their birth. There is obviously a disconnect between what a patient perceives a nurse to be and the actual value of the person at your bedside. You can even see this on social media when people post stuff like, "Oh, you're a labor nurse. Cool. I bet it's nice holding babies."
>
> **Fact:** *A good nurse can make (instead of break) your overall hospital experience.* A good nurse will believe she is assigned to advocate

for you. She has knowledge that you don't. She will evaluate your situation and can speak for you when you don't even know what needs to be said. Believe me, a good nurse is having conversations on your behalf unbeknownst to you.

Fact: *A good nurse wants to partner with you in your labor experience.* We literally have hearts to establish a relationship with you. We want you to trust us so we can partner WITH you during your labor experience, not do something TO you. This is why having the preconceived expectation that a labor nurse is your enemy is devastating to your hospital experience. You literally forfeit this entire chapter's value for your birth, and it will show when you are in postpartum evaluating your birth story. Establishing relationships is key, not only for the patient's experience, but for the safety of the birth as well.

Fact: *A good nurse can save yours or the baby's life.* She is at the bedside and will most likely be the first to recognize problems and will be the first to act. If you trust your nurse, you will be more at peace with the fluid changes of labor in general as your nurse acts on your behalf.

Fact: *A good nurse is your gift to navigating your mind and spirit as your birthing circumstances unfold.* A good nurse will be caring for your needs physically while evaluating how you are doing mentally and emotionally. Literally, as we are changing your position, caring about your comforts, keeping you clean, and changing your pads, we are listening to your fears, concerns, and answering your questions. This is establishing a relationship.

Now, to get to the place where you can help someone's mind and spirit, a relationship of trust has to already have been established. It is this same person who has given you water, cold cloths, toileted you, cleaned your perineum, addressed your pain, and provided for your physical needs who will have the privilege to speak as an emotional compass for you.

Some of my best moments with my patients have been after serving her needs physically and then a situation has needed a hard truth mentally or emotionally. Because she has trusted me physically to mean well for her, she can then be ready to trust me with something harder. I can pull up a chair, hold my patient's hand, look into her eyes, and tell her something she NEEDS to hear, while knowing it's not something she WANTS to hear. I can speak into my patient's spirit and help her recognize and cope with circumstances out of her control if she can trust me.

The paramount moment is when she trusts me and surrenders to that which is truly out of her control. It is then that she can proceed without fear, guilt, and shame and walk through the birth highlighting the positive of holding her healthy baby. Let me orient you to this person, your labor nurse, so you can begin to value her differently than the average patient.

KNOWING YOUR NURSE: THE TRAINING, THE JOB, HER BRAIN, HER HEART

The Training

Labor nurses are a tribe. Truly, I work with people who love pregnancy and the miracle of life, and that includes the male nurses in this discipline as well! We are a special breed of nurse, and our niche is delivering babies and all that comes with it. We are the literal face of the "hands-on" care experience at the hospital. Because this relationship is so important, I want you to have an idea of their training. All labor nurses are licensed medical professionals (registered nurses) who, through nursing school, have chosen this particular specialty.

The nursing school they graduate from can be through an AA program or through a traditional four-year bachelors of nursing route. Both routes will have the same hospital-hour requirement for the state in order to be an approved program that satisfies state regulations. Each state has a board of registered nurses or a state regulatory department that approves nursing programs, and each nurse will have to complete hospital-hour requirements in order to graduate.[2]

Once someone graduates from an accredited program in their state, they will consent to a background check and fingerprints. They will then need to pass a proficiency academic test in order to prove cumulative knowledge. In California, the Board of Registered Nursing requires a test called the NCLEX in order to get a license. Once passing, they get a license number and are required to renew it every two years from the state board. To keep a license, a nurse is required to complete thirty continuing education units in that two-year period and submit it to the state for renewal approval.

In addition to the regulatory requirements, some nurses will have acquired special certifications within the labor/delivery discipline. These special certifications reflect a nurse honing a particular skill set by pursuing education in an advanced way. Labor nurses can have special certifications in electronic fetal monitoring, breastfeeding, inpatient obstetrical care, postpartum care, or normal newborn care. Each one of these certifications requires continuing education to hold on to and must be actively pursued and reported to governing bodies.

Once licensed and hired, a new labor nurse will go through an orientation to the discipline of labor and delivery. They will be paired with an experienced nurse who will help them learn about labor, the operating room, recovering patients after delivery, and getting a feel for the unpredictability that comes with the job. It takes about six months of full-time work to learn just the discipline of laboring mothers, and skills like triage and high-risk patients will take more time.

The point I am trying to make is there is extensive education in the discipline of labor and delivery, and your nurse has spent a lot of hours honing the skills of her craft. She will bring all the experience of these hours of education into your labor room for the purpose of helping you have a fulfilling hospital birthing experience.

The Job

All labor nurses know how to deliver care across the sequence of the labor process. All labor nurses know how to admit a patient and be with them during their labor until delivery. They all know how to support unmedicated vaginal deliveries and also how to usher a medical patient through the labor process that requires more intervention. They can take care of healthy moms, diabetic moms, high-blood-pressure moms, and cesarean moms. All are the bedside eyes and ears of the physician and are trained to recognize and respond to that which is out of the norm. They know how to deal with unfolding elements that are within their scope of care and when to involve a collaborative effort with the attending physician. They also are the main person assigned to document your labor as it unfolds.

Most labor nurses will have skills in triage and can serve as the pregnancy ER of sorts. Some nurses will also work in postpartum and can alternate between labor areas and postpartum areas. Each labor nurse can bring to your room the skill set to perform the tasks delegated to this patient population. Each nurse will know how to contribute to the plan of care, take vitals, start an IV, give medications, and assess mother/baby on the monitor. Each can check your cervical dilation and labor progression, support you during an epidural, and be with you emotionally while you are in pain.

Her Brain

Most labor nurses have the ER-type brain where they love marching into a shift, not knowing what will come rolling through the door on any given day. Some days, you get a healthy mom having her baby and you get to partner with her during that pivotal day in her life. Other days, you see the cases that don't make the birthing videos and require intensive one-on-one care. Most labor nurses know the mundane can turn into an emergency quickly, and sometimes we don't get the "why" until after delivery. That means because your labor nurse has seen the possibilities of what can happen in labor, her mind is always working.

Sometimes things happen when we least expect it, so your nurse's brain is always working on planning for what's possible while excelling in the here and now. This means that during a casual conversation in your room, your nurse is listening to the fetal heart rate on the monitor, organizing loose cords, and moving chairs/tray tables out of the path from the bed to the door. They are always thinking about safety and making sure there is an escape route if we need to move quickly to the operating room. They are comfortable in the normal but also are trained for the traumatic case.

I want to tell you a hard truth. Every nurse knows this. Birthing floors of the hospital are usually the "happy" floor of the hospital. We have many great moments and good birth stories of welcoming life into the world. But often not talked about on mommy blogs is a truth anyone who has spent time with the general population in this discipline knows. The truth is if you do this long enough, you see the saddest of stories as well. Most nurses have stories that could scare you straight of what they have seen on the labor unit. They are not sharing these with patients, and I won't do that here either.

But I want you to know the hospital is a place where people go when they have problems, and that is just as true for birth as it is for anything else. I'm writing this for you to know what every single patient should know, things that are true for everyone. I'm not going to encourage you to google every ridiculous thing that could present itself in birth. I do want to make the point, however, that hospital nurses are the people who handle the sick, abnormal, and tragic cases, not just the normal healthy ones. Her brain is ready, and she will be a great resource for you if you know to value her; she will be a lifeline for the tragic case.

Her Heart

During nursing school, your nurse went through many hospital disciplines and saw many avenues of nursing. She chose labor because she was meant for it. The blood and mess that come with birth is not for everyone, and we all have our niche. Nurses in general have hearts to bring personal bedside care to their patient population and genuinely want to make a personal connection with you.

Believe me when I tell you, nurses value your thank-you cards and treats. We value it because it makes us feel like we made a connection that mattered for you on your big day. Your labor nurse loves the biology of pregnancy and birth, and the value of the miracle of life is usually not lost on her. We also have hearts to be a continual learner. I think most labor nurses I have known have team attitudes and teachable hearts.

Over the years, we have been taught to appreciate birth, and there are still a few deliveries that can bring me to tears if I have a chance to really know my patient's story. But I want you to know we have also learned to sit at the bedside of moms whose babies are in the NICU. We have supported moms who have had their baby transferred to a higher-care facility and are trying to deal with a new reality that didn't go according to plan.

We have counseled moms who come into triage and have endured physical abuse during their pregnancy. We have also learned to let our guard down and just cry with a mom who is holding her baby for the last time because his soul is already in the presence of God. We have prepared and walked tiny body bags to the hospital morgue, and it is a reminder that birth is not a perfect process and much is completely out of our control. We will try to bring peace to your situation no matter what it is and can help you through all the things that will be messy or complicated.

WHAT ELSE DOES A NURSE BRING TO YOUR BEDSIDE?

Your nurse will bring all of her *hospital* experience into your room with her when she cares for you. Let me tell you what else she will

THE *heart* OF A BIRTH PLAN

bring with her into your room. She will bring her own *life* experience into that room. Some nurses have walked the road of infertility and know a patient's struggle intimately who is trying to hold on to their in-vitro fertilization (IVF) pregnancy. Others have had unmedicated deliveries and know what it is like firsthand to deliver without an epidural. Some nurses have not had kids yet and are more objective, whereas other nurses might be biased about certain things due to their life experiences.

Some nurses have had medical emergencies themselves. Some have had cesarean sections. Some have had difficulty breastfeeding. Some have regrets about their birthing experiences and can help you to prevent making the same mistakes. Some have suffered fetal loss and know exactly what it is like to lose a child. Just as you are an individual with a certain personality and circumstance, so is your nurse. She will bring those experiences and personality base into your labor room. So, just as you, the patient, are coming into your birth room with your own personality and labor situation, your nurse is an individual coming in with her own makeup and experiences.

Your nurse will also bring her personality into your room with her. We all have personalities that will intersect with our education about labor and our personal experiences. We carry the same foundational training but will carry out our practice in a special unique way. Some nurses might be jokey with light personalities, while others are sticklers about doing everything "right" and may have less flexibility. Some are mercy oriented and will empathize with a patient in a deep personal way, while others have acute "unit awareness" and will be the first to help other nurses.

Some nurses are great detectives and have an uncanny ability to get to the bottom of a person's chart and will know things about their patient others wouldn't have found. Some are exceptional teachers and can explain things very well to their patients. Some are aggressive when advocating for patients, and others are more passive. Some will tell you hard truths while others will try their best not to offend you. All nurses will know the "tasks" of routine care, but each nurse will have their own care-delivery style. Your nurse is going to bring her personality into your room, and it probably will affect your care experience.

NURSE NIRVANA OR NURSE NIGHTMARE

Life gets interesting, and nursing nirvana occurs when you, the patient, get the perfect nurse for who YOU are! Just the opposite can be true. Not having a nurse who matches you can lead to an unfulfilling experience for both parties. If you want the "tell it like it is no matter what" lady as your nurse and you get a quiet, foot-massaging mercy-filled nurse, you may be annoyed. Probably what you needed was a nurse great at explaining things even when the truth is tough. The same thing is true the other way. If you are someone who needs a gentle, delicate communication style, you will probably be super annoyed by the "tell it like it is" lady who talks loudly.

If you are a patient who wants to be surrounded with less talking and just wants a room full of calmness, then you will be annoyed if you get a loud, detailed-oriented, policy-following nurse. She will flip on your lights and have loud discussions on the phone with the physician about your fetal monitoring strip while you are trying to harness your chi. All nurses are going to provide the same care for your vitals, monitor your baby, and understand your medications and other basics of the job. However, the perception of your care can be directly impacted by the correct matching of patient to nurse.

THE heart OF A BIRTH PLAN

If the nurse you are matched with does not match your needs, you can ask for a new nurse to be assigned to you. If it is not working for you as the patient, it probably is unfulfilling for the nurse as well. Nurse managers and charge nurses want you to have a positive birth experience, and if you have a specific delivery style in mind, it would be good to ask for it.

Please know specifically what you would need to define a good match though. Please don't ask for "anyone but that lady." Instead ask,

> "Could I have a calm nurse who explains things slowly so I can understand?"

> "Can I have a nurse who is patient with breastfeeding?"

These requests can easily be accommodated. A word of caution, however, if you are going to fire your assigned nurse: I have seen it many times where a match didn't seem like heaven at the beginning of the shift, but after labor unfolds, it turns out the nurse you didn't initially want becomes EXACTLY who the needs of the moment called for, becoming nurse nirvana for the patient in the end. Lastly, hospitals are full of humans, and humans are not perfect. Just as you are not your best while in labor, sometimes your nurse is having a bad day too. Be gracious when asking for a new nurse. She is human too.

We are all human with unique quirks. Each shift, when we are changing in the locker room before our shifts start, we are getting a view of the interpersonal dynamics on the labor unit that day. Sometimes, I giggle to myself as I see the patterns of a nuclear family or a church family on our nursing staff. There's always the quiet nurse, the loud one, the funny one, the one who has this idiosyncrasy or that one. It's literally just like your family reunion! We spend so much time together that we really learn so much about each other and live life's struggles with each other when we are not in your room, just like a quirky family.

I have to give you a word of truth my nurse family probably wouldn't tell you. Some of you will receive excellent care from nurses who are knee deep in their own life struggles. Outside of the hospital, we have loves and losses, families, and challenges just like anyone else does. When we are putting on our scrubs, we often are putting on our nurse hats while we are leaving and "putting off" the conflict with our husbands who remain unresolved, the strife of a wayward teenager, personal grief from a recent family loss, or our laundry list of mom stuff that will be there when our shift is over.

We put off regular life to care for you, and sometimes that experience is less than heavenly. Your nurse will not always be perfect because she is human. We honestly will try our best not to, but sometimes we bring excellence and imperfection to your bedside at the same time. Give a little grace, and kindly ask for a new nurse. It just may make your birthing experience all you were hoping it to be.

SPIRITUAL TRUTH—YOUR NURSE IS NOT SURPRISED BY LABOR IMPERFECTIONS

I want you to imagine me standing with my arms open wide. In my left hand, I am holding the hand of a pregnant woman. She is expecting problem-free scenarios, acquiescing nurses, limited intervention, undivided attention, maybe a pain-free experience, and a perfectly executed birth plan. Holding my other hand is a labor nurse. She is highly educated, has a wealth of experience, has been laboring mothers for ten plus years, and has seen it all.

She works in a place where it is evident that birth is an imperfect process, in an imperfect setting, with imperfect people, and probably will carry with it some level of pain or disappointment. She is assigned to help you. Can you see how these two people are coming from different places entirely? In order for the patient to perceive a positive birth experience, the surprise of imperfection has to be resolved. Most patients are surprised by what is completely normal to the nurse. Birth is not perfect. Labor and new life spring forth out of difficulty, pain, and the unexpected.

I see nurses every day coming alongside patients and gently easing them into the realities of imperfect situations. DAILY. I see nurses talking to patients who are crying in their rooms because when going to their regularly scheduled appointment they ended up needing to be induced for genuine medical reasons. Now, she is going to miss her baby shower because she got admitted to the hospital unexpectedly.

The nurses comfort her and talk to her about not being able to control it and how to move forward. I see nurses talking to their crying patients about feeling like a failure because they got an epidural or a cesarean section. I see nurses trying to explain to patients how a bad situation got great care and to hold a healthy baby is a great outcome. It is often nurses explaining to patients how the birth process is not perfect, and there are many variables along the way.

Nurses relate to patients as a guide by trying to set expectations right from when the patient is admitted. They know you don't know the imperfect parts. They will try to gently coach you through what to expect that is realistic and introduce imperfection to you slowly. What is normal for the labor process might be less than desired for the patient. Your nurse will lead you step by step as labor unfolds, sharing truths with you that will prepare you for what is next.

Standing at the bedside of my own patients teaching them about their own situations has brought the Genesis conflict front and center for me. Nurses may not always know it, but what they are coaching their patients about is actually a biblical, spiritual concept. In fact, I think if we can acknowledge the spiritual element, we can have these two people holding hands and understanding each other, thus creating a better hospital birth experience for you.

GENESIS CONFLICT: IS IT TWO OR THREE?

Let me explain how the Bible jumps off the page for me in this area. A long time ago, I went to a marriage church retreat, and the speaker (Alex Montoya) was stating over and over that we live in Genesis 3, not in Genesis 2. I don't remember a lot of anything else he said that weekend, but this basic biblical concept has never escaped me. In Genesis 2, there is the description of the first man and woman living and relating in a literally perfect world, in perfect relationship with Holy God.[3]

There is a profound absence of sickness, sin, offenses, mistrust, and death. There is only perfection. There is perfect relation to God, no brokenness, no addictions, no mistakes, no spiritual battle, and no enemies are introduced. I don't know what size Bible you have, but I have a big study Bible, and at only seven pages into a 2,500-plus-page Bible story, we get to Genesis 3.

In Genesis 3, we meet an enemy who offers a lie and a deception.[4] The famous forbidden fruit was eaten, and we have the first sin. Sin is the primary problem for the next 2,500-plus pages of the Bible, and with it comes human brokenness, suffering, sickness, death, and a fractured relationship with Holy God and each other. We live in

THE *heart* OF A BIRTH PLAN

Genesis 3, not in Genesis 2. It is so simple and yet so profound. We are married in Genesis 3. We raise children in Genesis 3 and are faced with the realities of a sinful imperfect world every day. We also are pregnant and give birth in Genesis 3, the broken place where pain exists and the undesired is possible.

Your nurse knows this. She may not always know the biblical origin of relational brokenness, or the spiritual introduction to sickness or death found in the Bible, but she can verify the fact that labor is rarely a perfect process and will try to usher this as truth to her patient. She sees Genesis 3 every day when it comes to birth.

Generally, the hospital is a setting where the sick suffer, situations can become serious, and bad things happen to good people. The spiritual truth of the sinful, imperfect world we live in is ever present in the discipline of labor and birth as well. Of course, it's our mission as doctors and nurses to try to minimize any bad experience and try to help any situation have a positive outcome. We are very good at it. Oftentimes, the hospital staff can protect you from knowing what you don't need to know in order to preserve your peace through changes in your labor. Your nurse has seen all of this, and she can guide you through any Genesis 3, imperfect birthing experience.

Somewhere along the way, though, expectant mothers are led to believe we give birth in Genesis 2, where there is no pain, danger, or medical diagnoses. There is a deception in some birthing classes that minimize the fallen-world possibilities. Most ladies come to the hospital expecting a Genesis 2 experience, and in most cases, it is the protected perfect idea that they have fashioned in their minds. It is completely unrealistic. Most ladies are shocked when they are confronted with the realities in the labor room, and I think it's because we are not preparing them to resolve their specific Genesis 2 perfect expectations.

SPIRITUAL ORIENTATION TO THE GENESIS SETTINGS

The Genesis story might be familiar to you, and even if you have never read it, you may know the synopsis as written above. Let's look at the main setting in the Garden of Eden before Genesis 3. Creation unfolds in an orderly fashion with human beings as the crown glory of the creation account as man is said to be made in the image of God.[5] To His image bearers, He gives dominion over the earth and the creatures inhabiting it.[6] God plants a beautiful Garden in Eden, and here He springs up "every tree that is pleasant to the sight and good for food."[7] Two trees are mentioned by name: the tree of knowledge of good and evil and the tree of life.

The Lord God puts man in the garden to work and keep the garden and to enjoy all of creation with one command. "You may surely eat of every tree of the garden, but of the tree of the knowledge of good and evil you shall not eat, for in the day you eat of it you shall surely die."[8] God doesn't want Adam to be alone, so He creates an equal counterpart, the woman Eve, to be his complement and helper in the Garden of Eden.[9] The man and woman enjoy a perfect relationship with one another, creation, and intimacy with Holy God. In fact, scripture even says they were naked and unashamed.[10]

Genesis 1 and 2 record a picture and life without sin, a relationship of man and wife delighting in each other without conflict and having a face-to-face relationship with God. They have dominion over creation, and taking care of it is a joy. God's creation exists in harmony until we are introduced to an enemy and sin in chapter 3.

A serpent, an enemy, approaches God's image bearers of creation and asks the woman a deceptive question. "Did God actually say, 'You shall not eat of any tree in the garden?'"[11] It is interesting to me that he asks Eve this specific question, because the command was given to Adam before her creation, which lends us to believe she may have only heard this directive through Adam and not God directly. It would seem from scripture she wasn't even there when this command was given originally. This leads her to doubt and question God as she decides whether or not she should eat from the tree of knowledge of good and evil.

The serpent promises, "You will not surely die. For God knows that when you eat of it, your eyes will be opened, and you will be like God, knowing good and evil."[12] She has a choice of whether to believe in God, even though she may be unsure, or trust her own judgment. She uses her best human judgment, and seeing that the tree looks good and can make one wise, she eats of it.[13]

She and Adam both eat and immediately are aware of their nakedness.[14] They try to cover themselves as they fear God seeing them now and try to hide from His presence.[15] Now they know shame for the first time and fear is introduced. When they are face-to-face with God, the man and the woman make excuses for their sin. The man blames his eating on the woman, and the woman blames her eating on the serpent who deceived her.[16] The consequences are great for the sin against God's only command in the garden. Consequences are given out to the serpent, woman, and the man.[17]

Now that the people are in a sinful state and will experience bodily death, God removes them from the presence of the tree of life, out of the garden of Eden. God does not want humankind to live forever in this sinful state and removes them from being able to eat from the tree of life.[18] Now instead of the image bearers guarding the garden, God places cherubim and a flaming sword to guard the way to the tree of life.[19] Adam and Eve's lives are changed because of human sin, and the humans know a very different life outside the Garden of Eden.

When I survey the scene of the world we live in, I see more in common with Genesis 3 about our lives, than Genesis 2. We live in a world where there is good and evil, and we have a will to choose what we value as truth. We live in a world with mortal people who, in their humanness, can offend others and cause pain. We also live in relationships often fractured by offenses, blame shifting, and yield pain due to our own sin or someone else's.

We can look around us and see we are living in a Genesis 3 arena where our mortalities are real, the human frame is frail, and in our human frames are unaware of what the future may hold. Also, the effects of sin and brokenness of this earth show itself through things like human poverty or sickness. In the animal kingdom, Genesis 3 shows itself by dominance and predation that is not present in Genesis 2. Even in our environments, we see things like earthquakes, floods, famine, and pestilence that remind us that the Genesis 3 earth has brokenness.

In fact, in the book of Romans, we see, "the whole creation is groaning together in the pains of childbirth" and creation itself is waiting to be restored to its Genesis 2 state.[20] "For the whole creation was subject to futility" waiting in hope for "creation itself to be set free from its bondage to corruption and obtain the freedom of the glory of the children of God."[21] The whole creation has been changed because of Genesis 3, and the earth itself awaits the day when it will be relieved of its struggles and sorrows.

YOUR GENESIS THREE HOSPITAL BIRTH

Expecting a Genesis 3 birth is letting go of the idea of perfection when it comes to birth and the labor process. Genesis 3 is a world where beautiful things exist, but it also can be hallmarked by brokenness. In the best of relationships, there are times of bliss and true beauty and also times of conflict or difficulty. It's just out there, both the beauty and the brokenness.

If you have been promised a Genesis 2 birth or are seeking a Genesis 2 birth, can I encourage you to face the reality that you don't give birth in the truths of page 7 of the Bible? You give birth in the other 2,500-plus pages. Be careful of the deception that nothing negative can happen in the experience of birth. Evaluate who is speaking into your spirit when it comes to birth. Birth has both the beauty and the brokenness of the world we live in. No one knows what your birth story will be, but it may not be perfect. The dream births do exist and are truly magical, but they come right next door to an imperfect situation in another room.

Your hospital experience of giving birth in an imperfect setting may be as simple as your nurse taking longer than you thought she should to answer your call light. It may be the room temperature not being to your liking. It may be your nurse being too loud. It might be the position shifts that are necessary, which you found annoying, due to your baby's heart rate. It might be you are fighting with your spouse during your labor. It might be the nurse having to adjust your belly monitor two thousand times during the night that got on your nerves. It may be the doctor you wish you didn't have or how complicated it is to sometimes just go to the bathroom with all the cords and the IV running. It may be that anesthesia wasn't available the second you decided on getting an epidural.

It may be the fact that sleeping is nearly impossible in the hospital. In fact, in postpartum, the imperfections of hospital life become evident with room visits. All the people who will visit your room while in postpartum will be surprising to you. In fact, they are all from different departments, and none of these visits will be coordinated with one another. You might notice as soon as the laboratory leaves your room after drawing your blood, the pediatrician will come in, then the birth certificate lady, and then the nurse. It may seem overwhelming, this parade of people before your discharge, but it is the imperfection that comes with the breed of hospital birthing.

Sometimes, the annoyances are labor events themselves, just natural biology. For example, it might be annoying to you that when your water breaks your body will continue to leak fluid until the baby comes. Most ladies don't expect this, and it can have the "gross" factor as your nurse helps you stay clean by changing your ginormous peripads. Labor itself can be imperfect as some people have painful contractions without cervical dilation. Others have fast labors and now have to detail and clean their car because the baby came in the parking lot! Some labors show interruptions in oxygenation on the monitor more frequently than others and will need more intervention based on these findings. Some ladies don't realize the pushing phase of labor is hard work and can last a few hours; it's unpleasant and usually not the dreamy birth plan.

If patients have a bad experience and have a bumpy ride through labor/birth, they can often try to look for someone to blame because they knew they didn't get perfection; they just don't know why. Blaming others is the hallmark of a Genesis 3 environment. Oftentimes, they falsely blame themselves, an intervention, the nurse, or the doctor because they don't know how to resolve the Genesis 2 versus Genesis 3 conflict. Letting go of the idea of perfection that is Genesis 2 and embracing the dual environment of Genesis 3, which is beauty with brokenness, is resolving this conflict.

Remember, home births and natural birthing education is for healthy mothers only without risk factors. I am mainly speaking to those who will give birth in hospitals. In the general hospital population of birthing mothers, we are seeing less of these healthy ladies. More often we are seeing mothers with obesity, diabetes, high blood pressure, and other factors. I believe that no matter what your diagnosis, we can highlight the beauty of your birth, while accepting the annoyances that come with a hospital birth.

Patients' acuities are changing, and we need to have you understand you will give birth in an environment with blood pressures, blood sugars, monitoring, and most likely medicine. We will be as mom/baby friendly as we can, but it's still beauty coupled with annoyances. To prepare your heart and spirit for a positive hospital birth experience, you must lay down your perfect expectations of Genesis 2 and open your spirit to be accepting of a Genesis 3 paradigm.

You will be given a Genesis 3 expert, called your nurse, who wants to partner with you so you can have as close to a dream birth as possible. But in order to appreciate your nurse and get all you can out of that relationship, you have to release yourself from perfection and be open to the birth adventure as it unfolds: the beauty and the brokenness. You have a great guide who can help usher you through your dreams into your reality, and her presence can lead you through any imperfection.

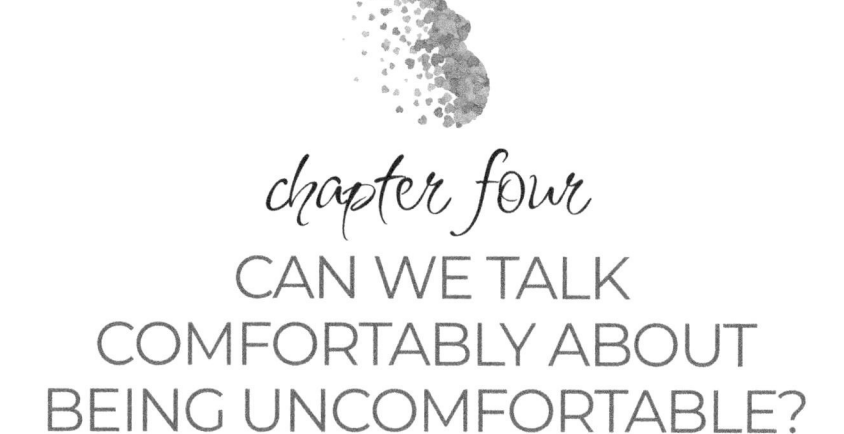

chapter four
CAN WE TALK COMFORTABLY ABOUT BEING UNCOMFORTABLE?

REALISTIC EXPECTATION IN GENESIS THREE HOSPITAL BIRTH: THERE WILL BE PAIN

The truth is labor and delivery can be the happy floor of the hospital. It also is the hospital home where pain resides. Real pain brings forth new life, again and again. It is an amazing concept really. As a bedside labor nurse, I have seen plenty of pain, front and center. Daily, nurses in labor units come alongside women in pain. It is a specialty in and of itself to be so comfortable in the presence of pain.

It actually is a great tightrope of sorts to walk: remaining sensitive enough to pain to want to help the person experiencing it but remaining calm enough in its presence to function as a provider with a clear head. There is so much I have learned about the concept of pain through doing this job, and I want to share with you what has jumped out at me.

When I think about preparing you for a hospital birth, addressing pain has to be the first thing some patients want to know about. Most people know the process of labor is uncomfortable, and most people assume the pain of uterine contractions is what I mean when I speak of the "pain of labor." Most people are surprised to know there are elements of pain or discomfort throughout the whole process of birth. In fact, anything that deviates from what you were "expecting" can be thought of as unpleasant. But there are actual physical realities I want you to be aware of if you are having a hospital birth, so you will not be surprised by these realities when you encounter them as part of your birth experience.

PHYSICAL ELEMENTS OF DISCOMFORT

When you come to the hospital triage, right away, you will be asked private questions and asked to remove all your clothing and put on a hospital gown. Some people are already uncomfortable with this. But during your triage time, in order to rule out active labor, and to determine if you should be admitted to the hospital, there will be a vaginal exam. Some first-time moms are experiencing this for the first time at the hospital, and others will experience it at the clinic during routine appointments toward the end of your pregnancy. The bottom line is the only way to determine if your contraction pattern is active labor is to check your cervix. One labor rule to remember: your cervix tells all.

We can see on the monitor if you are having contractions and how long they are lasting. We can physically look at you and determine if you are experiencing pain. But the only way to determine if your cervix is laboring is to feel it with a vaginal exam. Providers are trained to measure the cervix for dilation, effacement (thinning), and how high the baby is in your pelvis (station). Also with that same vaginal exam, providers are determining other characteristics of your cervix and whether the baby is presenting head down.

A non-laboring cervix will be harder to reach, thick, and has more of a firm piece of fruit feel. A laboring cervix will be softer, mushy, thinner, easier to reach, and dilated. The cervix is what will often determine whether or not you are admitted to the hospital. It is an important part of making decisions on the labor unit to manage someone's situation, and patients can find it uncomfortable. The definition of active labor is cervical change over time. So, you actually will be checked more than a few times during your labor to determine if plan of care is working and where you are in the labor process.

Other expectations that can cause discomfort during the hospital process can be when learning about inductions. Medical induction is a tricky thing because we are essentially asking your cervix to do something it isn't ready to do. If the cervix is not ready for labor, a medical induction can take days. Most people are not expecting that, and we see people coming in for their induction who bring everyone in the world and are expecting a baby by morning!

They are often disappointed when they realize it can take a day or two to even ready the cervix for receiving some induction methods. Inductions are the marathon of labor scenarios and can go on for a long time. Some patients get irritated with the process and are surprised that some methods of induction are uncomfortable.

Some people are grossed out at some of the realities of labor. For example, when your water breaks, the water will keep leaking out of your vagina until the baby delivers. Literally. Most of your amniotic fluid is baby urine along with water from the mother, and so it will keep being made and released once your bag is broken. Most ladies are surprised that even walking around the room they can leak fluid and in advance labor will need to be cleaned by their nurse. The amniotic fluid tells us a lot, and we look at the color and consistency of it as we are caring for you.

Some people are surprised to learn that IV medications are not the end all and be all of labor pain control. IV medications are given as a short-acting narcotic, like a dose of fentanyl. They will not take away all the pain of your contractions. Most people are expecting a miracle, and they discover that IV pain medication can help relax you through your contractions, but you will still feel the pain of your contractions. IV narcotics have limitations, and your nurse will review your fetal heart rate strip and determine whether delivery is imminent before administering these medications.

Other pain to be aware of when we are talking about birth is the pain of actual contractions themselves. This is what most people expect when we speak of labor pains. Most childbirth education is heavily into the physiology of birth and of coping with contraction pain. Any method of breathing techniques, visualization, Lamaze, hypnobirthing, etc. can help to cope with contraction pain. In my observations of laboring mothers with different philosophies of contraction pain control, they all can work.

The ones I see coping successfully seem to understand a few things. They understand to expect the pain, and although unpleasant, contraction pain is normal and safe. Fear and panic seem to intensify people's perception of pain. Reminding a patient that it has a beginning and an end can be helpful. Each contraction has a start and finish, and overall, the whole process has a beginning and will eventually end with the birth of the baby. Staying present in the moment has helped many mentally when coping with painful contractions.

THE DEPTH OF THE PAIN PROMISE

After working labor and delivery for a few years, a common biblical promise echoes in my mind while bedside with women going through very hard things in the arena of pregnancy and childbirth.

> "I will surely multiply your pain in childbearing; in pain you shall bring forth children."[1] | Genesis 3:16a

I am frequently reminded of the different ways pain presents itself as we get our "assignments" with unpredictable circumstances of labor and birth. The truth of birthing in Genesis 3 in a broken world is so evident, but the truth promised in Genesis 3 specifically to the woman about "in pain you shall bring forth children" has revealed the exponential possibilities of pain with pregnancy, birth, and new life that aren't the common "contraction" pain everyone assumes it meant.

People don't usually think of the many types of pain present, but let me show you how God has brought this verse to life for me over the years. Some women are pregnant with an unplanned and unwanted pregnancy and are coping with the decision to choose life. They may be scared, marginalized, rejected, and alone and are navigating being pregnant with these sources of pain.

Some people get their "assignment" of pain in the form of inability to conceive. Some start with suffering through accepting this harsh reality after many fertility treatments. Some conceive with IVF and have their own set of challenges. Some opt for surrogacy that presents its unique pain circumstances as well. Others may opt for adoption. There is pain in infertility, mentally, emotionally, and sometimes physically.

Some people conceive easily but have difficult pregnancies. Some have excessive vomiting as an actual condition and spend their pregnancy trying to keep food down enough to nourish themselves so they don't have to go to the hospital again for IV hydration and nutrition. Some have emotional grief during their pregnancies, like losing their mother or other family member who they wanted so badly to meet the baby. Some struggle with substance withdrawal as they try to do the best they can while pregnant but truly are in bondage to an addiction and can't quit. Others are coping with physically abusive partners during their pregnancy and are trying to figure out how to move forward for themselves and their baby.

There is also the pain of diagnosis. During pregnancy, many conditions can arise that will affect labor and birth. Some women find out they are gestational diabetic and have the challenge of altering their eating habits and pricking their fingers during the day. Some are hypertensive in pregnancy and are frustrated and disappointed they "have done everything right" and feel betrayed by their bodies.

Some are diagnosed with placenta previa and are adjusting to the reality of a cesarean section due to where the placenta attached itself, making vaginal delivery impossible. Some women are making peace with their diagnosis and are trading in natural birth plans for hospital-style medical ones. They try to make sense of things they never had control over in the first place as they grieve what might have been.

Some people have easier pregnancies and have difficult labors. There's the pain of actual contractions, which despite how much we desperately try to control pain, still exists. There's the pain of perineal tears and lacerations and postpartum cramping as your uterus goes back to its original size and shape. There's the pain of surgery, which we manage well, but leaves one in physical recovery and bears scars seen and unseen. There's the pain of emergent birth that forfeits the expectant birth plan altering the first few hours envisioned as a family because Dad wasn't able to be there for the birth and Mom is under general anesthesia. There's the pain of medically complicated deliveries such as hemorrhage that changes the patient's perception of birth because she came face-to-face with possible danger.

Then there are extreme assignments. There are those who will be told of fetal abnormality and will be faced with the pain of the unknown and difficult decisions. There are moms navigating their birth who now have the pain of leaving the hospital without their newborn because he/she is preterm or in the NICU for complicated reasons. Then there is the pain no one wants to talk about. It is rare, but it happens, and I'm not going to write a segment on pain without acknowledging the worst kind.

There is the pain of miscarriage or fetal demise with no medical explanation at all. While some mothers go home with emotional scars trying to make sense of all they had planned and prayed for going awry by simply getting a cesarean. There are others going home to empty nurseries and shattered dreams.

Not all ladies have all of these mentioned pain problems, of course. But over the years, watching the elements of pain and discomfort in this discipline has shown me truly God will not be mocked.[2] His promise of pain is true and three dimensional at times. The pain and discomfort scream of the brokenness of Genesis 3 life. Every lady will probably have something from this list that will challenge them physically, emotionally, or mentally through the process of labor and birth.

PAIN FROM OTHER WOMEN

There is another pain prominent, and it is the pain women give to other women. Nurses see it at the bedside on the daily. It is sad, but it is absolutely true. Mothers judge daughters for getting an epidural. Sisters laughing at sisters when they ask for pain medication. Family members and friends are upset with laboring mothers because they don't feel she's being "very strong." Mothers being judged for formula feeding by breastfeeding moms or even hospital staff. Even husbands and support people telling the nurse what to do for the patient when it comes to pain control. Every nurse has seen this. I have even seen a mother of a laboring mother ask me to withhold an epidural from the patient because she wanted her to be punished for an unwanted pregnancy. We don't do that, of course, but can I be honest with you?

As a labor nurse during the COVID pandemic, we worked through a time when visitors were restricted. Just the laboring mother and one other person were allowed in the labor and delivery area. Can I tell you how beneficial this was for the patient? Amazingly beneficial. Mothers-to-be were able to speak for themselves without any pressure from family and were able to construct their own best wishes for their delivery without fear of judgment or disappointing others. The mothers spent less time entertaining and performing for their family members and more time being present with their own style of birth.

The absence of visitors showed a remarkable positive difference for the laboring mother. My labor nursing advice is to consider limiting the voices speaking at your bedside during a hospital birth. If you want to moan through your contractions, then you should be able to moan without wondering what others might think about it! Moan away! If you want an epidural, then feel free to make that choice unencumbered by other women's opinions!

It might be to your own benefit to keep female expectations outside of your labor room. I wish I didn't have to say that, but it's true, and many nurses I work with have commented on how rested and relaxed the mothers were when limiting visitors was the policy. Since we have opened up again to one more visitor, allowing two at the bedside, we have once again seen a rise of external opinions affecting the laboring mother at the bedside. Mothers get pressure from the internet, social media, church friends, work friends, and especially family members. It's this pressure to be "super" right from the first contraction that is nuts and so unfair.

Somehow, the gold standard of being a woman I guess is having a natural unmedicated labor and birth and breastfeeding her baby without difficulty. I am so frustrated by this paradigm. You are not less than other women if you take IV pain meds or get an epidural. You are not to be shunned if you prefer to feed your baby a bottle. Most likely, if you got a cesarean section and your mother had a vaginal delivery, it's probably because you had a completely different set of circumstances! Women comparing themselves to other women or women on the internet promising perfection is crazy, and it is damaging in labor and birth.

I really feel for patients experiencing this type of pain and feeling like they "just didn't live up to what other women can do." It is false blame and false guilt that has no place in the birthing centers. I see women shift after shift, crying in postpartum because they are so upset at their perceived "weaknesses." I see women feeling like failures at birth, all the while cradling a healthy, beautiful baby! It actually is a huge reason why I wanted to write this book, because this type of pain is so pronounced.

I, too, wanted to be a part of the elite "natural birthing club." Because if that's your perception of a superwoman, who wouldn't want to be her? But that wasn't my assignment, and truthfully, I'm glad now I didn't have that type of birth. It makes me a better nurse to speak into the spirits of these women post-birth and truly help them see the truths of their labor circumstances, recognize what they never had control over, help them to release themselves from false guilt and blame, and really appreciate the healthy baby next to them.

UNINTENDED VISITOR PAIN

In postpartum, the absence of many visitors during the pandemic was beneficial for the baby as well. Mothers had time to spend skin to skin with their babies. Breastfeeding was uninterrupted and more peaceful. Mothers were actually getting a few hours of rest in postpartum. Previously, we saw mothers interrupting breastfeeding to let family members hold the baby and be passed around the room. Letting the family come into labor units has a consequence.

I worked the night shift for many years. Patients would spend their day in postpartum entertaining visitors and letting everyone hold their baby. They wouldn't rest at all and often, because of appearances, would not even care for themselves properly. Because who wants to walk around and change their bloody pads in a hospital gown in front of family? They would put off toileting, breastfeeding, and even napping in order to not offend family. Then, when everyone would go home, they would be left with a crying baby at their bedside, having a hard time breastfeeding, and the mothers would start crying.

They were actually mentally and physically exhausted. They hadn't prioritized caring for themselves and now are breaking down in the middle of the night, understandably. Now, let's consider a cesarean patient or a two-day medical induction patient. Their body has been put through a marathon of work, and they literally have physical recovery to do. Visitors are doing an injustice to these patients, and the patient will not show that to the family because "superwomen" don't hurt family feelings. But trust me, they are paying for it at 3:00 a.m. when the wheels come off. It's then, when family isn't there, that she feels free to let go and be emotional. It is the nurse who will try to help this lady get some self-care and some much-needed rest.

My advice: bring one very helpful person to the hospital with you who is interested in only honoring your wishes and is great with change. While you are in labor, you may be your nurse's only patient and may have her undivided attention. You also might share your nurse with another patient for a time. But mostly, you will have her at your bedside a lot! That is not the case in postpartum. Your nurse will be assigned up to four mother-and-baby couplets in postpartum. That's eight humans requiring things from one nurse! This is when a helpful visitor becomes paramount.

Your nurse will need to prioritize care to fresh surgical patients and medically complicated patients. If you have someone competent at your bedside to change the baby's diaper and hold the baby so

THE *heart* OF A BIRTH PLAN

you can sleep for two hours, it will make a world of difference for a breastfeeding mother. Please bring someone who will help you in postpartum. It is not helpful to you to bring someone who is going to sleep in the visitor bed the entire time and not help you with baby care. This is a recovering time but also a transition to being able to care for yourself at home. Your nurse will not be at the bedside as often in postpartum.

PROMISE OF PHYSICAL DELIVERY—YOU WILL BE DELIVERED FROM YOUR PAIN

Through this promised pain, you will have a nurse assigned to care for you who can understand your particular pain and meet you right where you are in your labor journey. Nurses are comfortable sitting next to someone in pain and evaluating whether the pain is normal and safe pain, like contractions, or anxiety/panic pain that needs to be addressed in other ways. Nurses can guide you into the best pain management for your situation.

If your situation is high blood pressure, your nurse knows an early epidural will help tremendously with your pressures, labor experience, and will help to prevent seizures. If you are having panic attacks and anxiety, your nurse can address this pain in a different way by talking with you and helping you take things one step at a time instead of being overwhelmed with the whole experience at once.

Your nurse can accommodate many different styles of pain control, such as hypnobirthing, breathing techniques, and other modalities. As long as the nurse can monitor your baby safely for your situation and your desires fall within hospital policy (i.e., no open flames), then your preferences can be honored. There are two things your nurse will speak to if they occur. First, if there is ever an issue of safety, she will speak up and let you know. Second, she has the experience to know when laboring can become suffering. Laboring is safe pain with progression. Suffering is pain that is not progressive and needs a change. If she sees you move into suffering needlessly, then she will speak up. She will suggest appropriate interventions.

For example, if I have a patient who really wanted a natural delivery but has been stuck at 7 cm for hours and is becoming frustrated, I will intervene. If I examine her and she has more cervix on one side than the other, I might suggest lying on the side with the cervix and maybe adding a half dose of fentanyl to relax through the next thirty minutes of contractions. If the patient will try it, I have seen it work and patients can change to completely dilated quickly after mixing it up a bit. Your nurse has this type of knowledge and may have some tips, tricks, or suggestions that may be just what you need at the right time. For labor pain control, there are usually ways we can help you if you are open to receiving it.

THE DELIVERY

The pain of labor contractions will have a start and an end. It has an assigned set of time and will not go on forever. *The promised end is the delivery of your baby.* Nurses literally say in the hospital when we are calling the doctor "We are ready for delivery in room 321." Delivery is the promised end to the waves of contractions. During your time in labor, you will be challenged with being in an uncomfortable situation, and it will reveal how you cope with circumstances out of your control.

You won't know how many contractions you personally will have to feel before your release from it, and each person is different. Each labor pain will challenge you to fight the urge for fear and control and to release yourself in your spirit. But the whole challenge of your labor comes with the physical promise of delivery from it.

LABOR ANALOGY TO SPIRITUAL DELIVERY

Just as it is the truth that you will be physically delivered from the pain of contractions, the physical becomes a picture of the spiritual. I believe God has given me this heart's desire to lean into the concept of childbearing in the Bible because I see its truth at the bedside. Bible knowledge echoes in my mind sometimes when I call a physician for delivery. I am not a seminary scholar, but I have been studying the Bible for twenty-plus years, and some ancient truths speak of deliverance that warrant attention.

The definition of deliverance is salvation.[3] The definition of *salvation* is "the state of being saved or protected from harm" or in theology "the deliverance from the power and penalty of sin; redemption"[4] In the physical reality of childbirth, the painful contractions come to an end with "delivery." The delivery marks the end of the contractions and labor itself. The Bible references childbearing pains many times, referring to the physical act of birth. When the Bible uses childbirth as an analogy, it describes a period of suffering marked with an ending of deliverance. Since everyone in any generation can picture a woman in labor, the picture can serve as an analogy for something deeper.

Delivery for Israel

In the Old Testament, the nation of Israel has a special relationship with God. He reveals Himself to the people of Israel and teaches them about the relationship between people in Genesis 3 and Holy God. The people are given what they must do to worship God and follow Him. Summarizing the whole Old Testament stories: the people follow God for a time, then go their own way. They endure consequences for not following God as a nation and endure many hardships that could have been avoided. When God sends prophets to them to describe warnings before the consequences are enacted, the prophets sometimes speak in this childbirth analogy.

> Now why do you cry aloud? Is there no king in you? Has your counselor perished, that pain seized you like a woman in labor? Writhe and groan, O daughter of Zion, like a woman in labor, for now you shall go out from the city and dwell in the open country; you shall go to Babylon. There you shall be rescued; there the LORD will redeem you from the hand of your enemies.[5] | Micah 4:9–10

In fact, these people were taken from Jerusalem into Babylonian captivity as prophesied.[6] They spent seventy years in captivity and then, as promised, were delivered. In 538 BC, Cyrus King of Persia fulfills the prophecies that the captives would be freed.[6] This account verified in the book of Ezra shows the words, "and the LORD stirred up the spirit of Cyrus, King of Persia" for him to send God's people back to Jerusalem.[7]

God promises delivery to His people Israel. God is not finished with His people of Israel, even today. There are many promises to them that are still future to us now. Their time of suffering in Genesis 3 will end with delivery as promised in the books of Daniel and Revelation.

Delivery for Each Person in Their Personal Relationship to God

When we last looked at Genesis 3, our Adam and Eve, due to the penalty of their sin, are outside the presence of God. They are to work the land in toil and hardship and will experience eventual death:

> And to Adam he said, "Because you have listened to the voice of your wife and have eaten of the tree of which I commanded you 'You shall not eat of it,' cursed is the ground because of you; in pain you shall eat of it all the days of your life; thorns and thistles it shall bring forth for you; and you shall eat the plants of the field. By the sweat of your face you shall eat bread, till you return to the ground, for out of it you were taken; for you are dust, and to dust you shall return."[8] | Genesis 3:17–19

All of initial creation is broken, in a sense, laboring away in the pain of the Genesis 3 curse in our everyday lives. However, tucked away in the verses of Genesis chapter 3, right before the promise of pain in childbirth for the woman, are the words of God speaking to the enemy, a promise of human deliverance.

> "I will put enmity between you and the woman, and between your offspring and her offspring; He shall bruise your head, and you shall bruise his heel."[9] | Genesis 3:15

This is known as the first promise in the Bible that prophesies deliverance. This deliverance is our release from the Genesis 3 curse of bondage to sin. Throughout our lives on this earth, each of us will wrestle with good and evil desires within us in our human frame. The imperfect state of humans, our sinful state, does not allow for us to enjoy direct relationship with Holy God. God has a plan for redemption from the toil of the human sinful state. The promise is called the Gospel, or promised Good News for humanity. The heart's belief in Jesus Christ's perfect life, death, and resurrection is the bridge back to direct relationship with Holy God.

This is the designed plan for human redemption. The first time the promise is mentioned is here. This verse is the first stitch sewn into the Bible and weaved through the entire Old Testament, pointing to an eventual Redeemer who would come to crush the enemy and free captive sinners from this Genesis 3 curse. To be released and redeemed from our sin is the plan to restore our uninhibited relationship with God. The Redeemer, the Great Physician, will be called on for "delivery."

God has a plan for spiritual delivery for any man/woman wanting to be relieved from their sinful state and enjoy a relationship with God personally. This invitation is open to all people now. People of today can now be delivered from a broken relationship to God by embracing God's plan for spiritual delivery.

God's Plan for Delivery to a Genesis Three Earth

God also plans on delivering this Genesis 3 groaning earth. In a time future to us, the Bible promises to renew the earth. Isaiah describes a time in which sin is absent, and even the animal kingdom is returned to a Genesis 2 state:

> The wolf shall dwell with the lamb, and the leopard shall lie down with the young goat, and the calf and the lion and the fattened calf together; and a little child shall lead them. The cow and the bear shall graze; their young shall lie down together; and the lion shall eat straw like the ox. The nursing child shall play over the hole of the cobra, and the weaned child shall put his hand on the adder's den. They shall not hurt or destroy in all my holy mountain; for the earth shall be full of the knowledge of the LORD as the waters cover the sea.[10] | Isaiah 11:6–9

Just like physical labor, the time for pain will be followed by delivery. God's people will live in Genesis 3 for a prescribed time, and then God's people will be delivered. God proposes a Messiah, a Deliverer, to take away our sins and make us ready for personal relationship with Holy God again. We can be redeemed from our sin and have a new way of relating to God personally. Even the time for earth and creation to remain in a broken Genesis 3 state is fixed.

There will be a certain amount of time allotted. It will not be forever. God's redemptive plan will follow the pattern of pain of a laboring mother. The time of laboring will be followed by a time of delivery, and the Bible describes it many times: delivery from pain, delivery for His people, and ultimately delivery for all of creation.

chapter five
LISTENING BETWEEN THE HEARTBEATS AND HEARING YOUR SPIRITUAL TRUTH

WHAT I'M TRAINED TO LISTEN FOR

The hallmark sound of any hospital labor room is the electronic fetal heart monitor. It's galloping steady beats are the conversation being had between any labor/delivery nurse and your baby. Nurses are trained to listen to the electronic fetal monitor pulse as they are doing other things while in the room, always having an ear on the rhythm. We are just trained to "listen and do."

Nurses have an ear on that fetal heart rate as they are asking your admission questions, starting your IV, taking your vitals, and even while conversing with you at the bedside. We can't see your baby with our eyes before he/she is born, but I assure you we already have a relationship with them. During your care, we are responding to the cues your baby gives through the pattern of that fetal heart rate and rhythm. Believe it or not, that pattern and rhythm tell us so much about your baby.

A few beats here and there is not enough to evaluate the baby's rhythm, but even just twenty minutes of continuous tracing of that heart rate can tell me a whole lot! I can learn if your baby is well oxygenated, neurologically sound, and determine a baseline rate. Fluctuations from that baseline rate will give me information as to how the baby is tolerating labor.

I look for fluctuations that are measured to show me your baby is oxygenated and the sympathetic and parasympathetic nervous systems are intact and harmonious. I can hear fluctuations that are cluing me into the interruptions in oxygenation that will need my recognition and intervention to resolve during labor. The fetal heart rate can also give me clues as to how the mother is doing. It can show me a possible brewing fever or a dehydrated mother. It's an amazing thing really.

Listening, interpreting, and acting on that fetal rhythm is a huge part of the nurse's job. Your baby will even be on a central monitoring system so every nurse on the unit can see every strip on the unit at all times. We listen, look at your strip continually, and chart anywhere from hourly to as frequent as every fifteen minutes or more often, depending on your stage of labor and the quality of your tracing.

After years at the bedside, I started to realize that patients were communicating their hearts to me, too, not in words usually, although verbal communication is part of it. When I started listening to what patients were saying and mostly what they were NOT saying, it became evident to me that I was listening between the fetal heartbeats into the screaming silence of the spiritual angst of my patients.

One interaction with my patient doesn't give me enough information, but after spending hours and hours at the bedside with someone, I realize they have a spiritual heart rhythm they are communicating to me. There is actually a spiritual posture each patient has that determines how I interact with them, the quality of our relationship, and it ultimately affects their perception of whether or not they have a good birth experience. Now, the spirit you bring to the hospital room is as loud to me as that heart rate on the monitor. Let me tell you what I have learned and how it can help you.

HERE'S WHAT I HAVE SEEN

I have seen laboring women for years. I have seen women in great pain using their best manners to thank me for changing their pads and keeping them clean. I have seen women yelling and screaming at their husbands/significant other through labor. I have seen patients afraid of medical care, refusing help, and throwing monitor parts on the floor. I have watched mothers cry over the joy of seeing their babies for the first time, moving me to tears myself that birth can be so beautiful. I have seen patients screaming their heads off sending chills down the spines of people innocently walking down the hallways. I have seen women kicking and punching the hospital bed rails.

I feel like I have seen every birth plan known to man, some reasonable, some cultural, some creative, and some scary. I have seen teenage mothers come in with little to zero education of how the baby is even going to physically come out of their bodies, and I have seen them breeze through labor. Conversely, I have seen labor nurses tremble and cry when they themselves need a cesarean section because they have seen too much and their education betrays them in the patient bed.

I have seen how different cultures handle pain—and there *is* a difference! I have been punished by patients who didn't like their experience by things like giving me the silent treatment or complaining about normal procedures for their situation, such as needing a catheter. I have also seen the sweetest couples dealing with the deepest tragedies somehow with a peace that inspires awe.

All of these behaviors boil down to two presenting spiritual rhythms. Presented with the reality that labor tends to reveal, patients realize they are not in control. Patients come to a crossroads where they must decide how to deal with their fear and anxiety if they are not in control of their circumstances. If left unchecked, the spirit of fear will progress to what I call a spirit of resistance. Or the patient will yield to a spirit of surrender, which is marked with a spirit of peace through the pain that can partner with her caregiver.

EXAMINING THE SPIRITUAL POSTURE OF RESISTANCE

The characteristics of a spirit of resistance vary, but mainly there is an element of fighting the process of birth as a whole. People express this differently as they are trying to cope with an uncomfortable situation they have realized is mostly out of their control. The inability to cope with fear and anxiety in their spirit when their circumstances are unpleasant and out of their control reveals a spirit of resistance.

There are those who resist the idea of physical pain. They can be the patients who are tensing up through contractions and fighting the labor process of their own bodies. These can also be the patients who are seen being blatantly resistant by being violent or loud: kicking, screaming at people, grabbing nurses, or thrashing around. A person laboring in this manner will accentuate each contraction, tend to experience more pain, and those labors can be longer and arrested.

Some people think when I say resistance, I am referring only to people who are intent on natural birth plans in contrast to people who are more medically minded and want greater pain control. This is not just about natural birth plans void of intervention, although rejecting advice, help, and intervention from an educated nurse is definitely a type of resistant spirit. However, the opposite is true as well. When a medically minded patient comes to the hospital in pain, they may be expecting immediate pain control.

There are ladies who ultimately resist the idea of feeling any pain at all, and when they demand an epidural in triage, they panic when they discover an epidural is a process over time. With this unmet expectation of a pain-free experience, they panic, give way to fear, and end up with a resistant spirit of anger and perceive poor care.

Some ladies literally sign refusal-of-treatment forms to display their spirit of resistance. Some will shut down when things don't go their way, refusing to answer the nurse's questions or giving the silent treatment. There are some who refuse ultimate truths like needing a cesarean section for genuine reasons. In desperate attempts to maintain control over something, some patients try to control the hospital staff with their requests. Some reject suggestions by the nurse that can actually lead to unnecessary suffering. Some reject monitoring restrictions, are noncompliant with diagnosis treatments like blood sugars for diabetics, or even have spotty prenatal care because of their resistant spirit.

COSTS OF A RESISTANT SPIRIT

The spirit of resistance is detrimental to your hospital experience. If you labor with a spirit of resistance, you forfeit the blessing your nurse can be for you in triage, labor, and postpartum. Resistant patients do not bond with their nurses and have a hard time perceiving their hospital experience as positive. They are the patients who most often call the nurse, have unrealistic expectations, treat staff poorly, and in postpartum have an aura of anger about their birth.

Oftentimes, this is not correlated to poor care but to a perception of poor care due to a resistant spirit. In fact, I have seen resistant patients in situations where the medical team has literally saved the lives of mother or baby. But in postpartum, this exact patient will describe her birth experience to her family members as a terrible hospital experience. In truth, they were unable to cope with the circumstances of their particular birth spiritually and correctly adapt to that which was out of their control.

As a provider at the bedside, when I encounter a resistant patient, I am limited in the ways I can truly help her. If you refuse my care, explanations, education, and suggestions, then figuratively, you tie my proverbial hands behind my back. You change me from a guide to help and bond with you to someone reduced to acquiescing to your pillow-fluffing suggestions. You will isolate yourself to labor alone and will forfeit the nurse/patient relationship that can be such an asset to your experience.

Resistance is hallmarked by fear and control and will always set up the provider as the enemy or the annoyance. If I am the enemy or the annoyance, then there is a chasm between us, and our relationship is meaningless. The thing about labor is once it starts, it will carry through until completion, regardless of how well you are coping. If you labor with a resistant spirit, your labor can change to needless suffering, and your nurse will be reduced to an innocent bystander to your palpable feelings of abandonment. No wonder why you will perceive a negative birthing experience!

EXAMINING A SPIRITUAL POSTURE OF SURRENDER

When we are talking about the heart of a birth plan, the true center, this section is the most important part of this book. Please believe me, understanding the spiritual posture of surrender is the key element to a fulfilling birth. The complete opposite of a resistant patient is one who has a spirit of surrendered submission. Not surrendered and submitted to me, or the doctor, but to the labor process as a whole. There is a silent acknowledgment of a painful process that ends when it culminates in the birth of the baby.

A surrendered patient has made her peace with her labor "assignment" and knows her spiritual truth of who is in control. Ultimately, she knows events will unfold, medical people will respond, and her desires will have little effect on her circumstances. She will labor willingly in Genesis 3, an imperfect setting, with imperfect people, and will most likely experience discomfort along the way. She believes and trusts in her guide, the nurse, and is flexible with position changes and nursing care and is willing to take suggestions.

Her spirit of submitted surrender is hallmarked by the ABSENCE of the need to control and the freedom and erasure of fear. She will make relational connections with her nurses. A natural-minded patient will have a higher chance of her birth plan becoming her reality with a peaceful acceptance of pain, adequate coping skills, and an aura of surrender. Medically minded patients will describe equally positive birthing experiences by surrendering to the process of medical procedures, epidurals, and protocols in place for their particular diagnosis.

In postpartum, these are the people who most likely will report thanks to their nurse, appreciate the outcome of their beautiful baby, and live free of judgment and false guilt. They will be able to report a good experience, even if there are undesired outcomes, like the baby needing care in the NICU or difficulty in the postpartum period. Submitted surrender is a beautiful thing. In fact, it is a biblical thing. The most important part of your birth plan is to reach ultimate spiritual surrender. It is only with spirited surrender you will look back on your birth story appreciating the blessings along the way, even in a tough birth.

BEDSIDE COACHING

If I have patients who are resistant, I will try to usher them to a more surrendered spirit as much as they will allow. I start by reminding them that discomfort is normal and safe. I will encourage them to embrace relaxation through the pain over panic and help them take one contraction at a time. I will remind them they are not alone. I will remind them they didn't do anything wrong, and change is normal with the birth process if variables come their way. If they can appreciate the uniqueness of their own story and love themselves through it, they are more likely to have a better birth. I try to make that happen as much as possible at the bedside.

But it's always better to have a patient surrender before they arrive in the labor unit, because trying to teach someone in pain is not normally easy. In order for you to come to your birth truly spiritually submitted, there are a few things I would say to do beforehand.

The Heart of Your Birth Plan

1. Think of every detail you dream of for your birth. Write down how you want it to go.

2. Now, evaluate honestly: Would you be okay if you didn't get ANY of those things, but you had a beautiful healthy baby?

3. Acknowledge that each piece of information about your pregnancy is forming your unique birth scenario, and most of it will be out of your control.

4. If you can't predict your labor situation and you can't control it, then you can release yourself from blame or false guilt beforehand. We want to be fair to ourselves, and it is loving to yourself to tell yourself the truth.

5. Move forward into the unknown of your labor experience with a spirit of surrender to the process and enjoy the gifts

along the way, like forming meaningful partnerships with your nurses and holding your beautiful baby.

BIBLE COACHING: SPIRITUAL CONCEPT OF THE GARDEN, A DIFFERENT GARDEN

I've told you the part I can truly say in hospital scrubs at the bedside. Now, let me tell you what I can say here in my own writing. The spiritual heart of your labor is the ability to go to your "garden." Your ability to go to the garden is the key to spiritual surrender. Let me explain.

This is a new garden, not the Garden of Eden where sin was born, but the Garden of Gethsemane. The Garden of Gethsemane is a place in the Bible where Jesus Christ, hours before He was betrayed by a close companion, teaches us a prayer posture. The story takes place the night before His crucifixion. Something amazing and new to humanity was about to take place. Jesus in the Garden of Gethsemane shows us how He prepared His heart for the carrying of His cross. It was a heart's preparation for a physical and spiritual assignment, His cross.

There is a popular casual phrase in Christianity we can say off the cuff, and it usually sounds something like: "It's my cross to bear." Usually in the United States, if people are saying this, they might be referring to things like a tough boss, a difficult relationship, or the inability to lose weight, amongst other common displeasures. Some people refer to a "cross to bear" as something they would rather not have but have accepted it isn't going anywhere. Some people actually say this phrase in sarcastic jest to their situation, but it is an actual reference to a directive in scripture describing how to follow Jesus as recorded by Luke, Matthew, and Mark:

──────LUKE──────

Then he said to them all: "Whoever wants to be my disciple must deny themselves and take up their cross daily and follow me."[1] | Luke 9:23, NIV

──────MATTHEW──────

Then Jesus said to his disciples, "Whoever wants to be my disciple must deny themselves and take up their cross and follow me."[2] | Matthew 16:24, NIV

──────MARK──────

Then he called the crowd to him along with his disciples and said: "Whoever wants to be my disciple must deny themselves and take up their cross and follow me."[3] | Mark 8:34, NIV

This is a three-part directive, and it is all demonstrated in the Garden of Gethsemane. First, one must deny herself. Second, she must be ready to take up her cross. In Jesus's case, it was a literal cross for crucifixion; in our case, it's going to be our labor assignment for the application. After the heart is right in steps one and two, a person is truly biblically surrendered to their God-given assignment, and in step three, will follow Jesus in their individual circumstance. I believe the story of Jesus in the Garden of Gethsemane shows the true heart of someone submitted to the will of God.

The meaning of "taking up your cross" to a person in Jesus's time period is completely different from the appropriations we make today.[4] This isn't talking about a simple annoyance. A first-century person listening to Jesus say this is going to apply what they know of "a cross." These people watched as Romans forced people to carry their own execution device to the place where they would die the most torturous, painful, and humiliating death possible.[4] The cross didn't represent something of spiritual freedom, grace, forgiveness, or anything positive we may attribute to it today.[4] It only represented a gruesome, gory death that no one in their right mind would want to go through.[4]

Quite simply, the call is to deny yourselves, take up the cross, and follow Jesus. What does it mean to deny yourself? I believe it can look different for everyone in different situations. Jesus asked simple fishermen who were casting their nets into the sea, "Follow me and I will make you fishers of men."[5] In order to be Jesus's disciples, scripture says they immediately left their nets to follow Him. Sometimes, you may have to leave that which you *know* to follow Jesus.

The gospels of Matthew, Luke, and Mark all share the story of a rich young ruler who approached Jesus asking what he must do to inherit eternal life. The man was certain he was religious enough to have followed all the commandments. As Mark records,

> Jesus looked at him and loved him. "One thing you lack," he said. "Go, sell everything you have and give to the poor, and you will have treasure in heaven. Then come, follow me." At this the man's face fell. He went away sad, because he had great wealth.[6] | Mark 10:21–22, NIV

He went away sad because he loved his life and was not willing to lay his riches down to be a disciple of Jesus. Sometimes, you may have to leave that which you *love* to follow Jesus. He wants your heart. It doesn't have to be something sinful in your life for God to ask you to lay it down. What God is always asking you to lay down is your will (what you know, what you want, or what you love) and exchange it for His. Lay down your plans to truly follow what He has planned for you. He is still asking that of believers today. But what I have learned over the years is laying down your will in some instances might be a gentle laying down of something you wanted or what may be familiar. Other times, it is much more like crucifying your will because it hurts to let it go.

Denying yourself what you wanted and prayed for and exchanging it for God's plan is like watching what you wanted most going to its death. It is your will that must be crucified, put to a gruesome bloody death. And if you are crucifying your will to follow Christ, there will be some pain involved. It's going to hurt to lay it down, to truly be willing to say, "This is what I want most with my whole heart, but I want You more. If this is not Your plan for me, I choose You. I choose to trust You, believe You, and know You will walk with me in whatever You have for me." This is true biblical spiritual surrender, and it is hard even for the seasoned Christian.

For the purposes of your labor, it might mean acknowledging you want a vaginal delivery more than anything else, but you are willing to lay this down if the need arises. It may mean not wanting monitoring more than anything else, but you are willing to go with it if your baby shows it might need more monitoring to be safe. It may mean not wanting an IV, but you are willing to have an IV in case of emergency situations.

It may mean wanting a quick epidural but being okay if the anesthesiologist is taking care of another patient at the same time as your request. It may mean you wanted delayed cord clamping for the baby but being okay in your spirit if the baby requires resuscitation. Whatever your labor assignment becomes, true biblical surrender is having an internal spirit of peace as your labor circumstances unfold, your "cross" if you will.

But how do we get here to this place of true biblical surrender, the heart of it all? Most people skip to the cross-carrying part of their lives without really doing the hard work of denying and crucifying their will, which can leave them in a spirit of resistance. We must convert from a spirit of resistance to a spirit of surrender to truly walk in our Genesis 3 assignments glorifying God. If you are a believer in the Bible, I am dying to share with you how God has highlighted the important spiritual work of what I call "going to the garden." The gospels of Matthew, Mark, and Luke all record Jesus going into the Garden of Gethsemane before the carrying of His cross.

YOU MUST GO TO THE GARDEN BEFORE CARRYING YOUR CROSS

After the last supper and before His betrayer found Him for arrest, Jesus goes to the Garden of Gethsemane to pray. This time of prayer is recorded in three gospels.

---MATTHEW---

> Then Jesus went with his disciples to a place called Gethsemane, and he said to them, "Sit here while I go over there and pray." He took Peter and the two sons of Zebedee along with him, and he began to

be sorrowful and troubled. Then he said to them, "My soul is overwhelmed with sorrow to the point of death. Stay here and keep watch with me."

Going a little farther, he fell with his face to the ground and prayed, "My Father, if it is possible, may this cup be taken from me. Yet not as I will, but as you will." [7] | Matthew 26:36–39, NIV

―――――― MARK ――――――

They went to a place called Gethsemane, and Jesus said to his disciples, "Sit here while I pray." He took Peter, James and John along with him, and he began to be deeply distressed and troubled. "My soul is overwhelmed with sorrow to the point of death," he said to them. "Stay here and keep watch."

Going a little farther, he fell to the ground and prayed that if possible the hour might pass from him. *"Abba*, Father," he said, "everything is possible for you. Take this cup from me. Yet not what I will, but what you will."[8] | Mark 14:32–36, NIV

―――――― LUKE ――――――

Jesus went out as usual to the Mount of Olives, and his disciples followed him. On reaching the place, he said to them, "Pray that you will not fall into temptation." He withdrew about a stone's throw beyond them, knelt down and prayed, "Father, if you are willing, take this cup from me; yet not my will, but yours be done." An angel from heaven appeared to him and strengthened him. And being in anguish, he prayed more earnestly, and his sweat was like drops of blood falling to the ground.[9] | Luke 22:39–44, NIV

This has long been one of my favorite passages, and Luke's writing as a physician has captured my attention. It is my favorite passage because it shows the humanity of Jesus as He is about to face His God-given assignment. It shows the human emotions we identify with as we walk in Genesis 3 in painful circumstances and how Jesus goes straight to the Father with them. It shows a correct prayer posture of surrendered submission we can emulate in our own assignments here on earth, your labor included.

In the Garden of Gethsemane, note:

1. Jesus prays ALONE. He is with His group of disciples, but for this type of prayer, He goes farther and farther away from them to be alone with the Father during this type of garden prayer. *Sometimes there is no substitution for genuine, earnest private prayer.*

2. Jesus's posture is falling on the ground, pouring out all of His human emotions, and is greatly distressed and troubled. Luke even records He was in agony while praying. His sweat became "like great drops of blood falling to the ground." *Bringing your emotions to the garden prayer is welcomed. God welcomes the truth of your heart naked and bare before Him.*

3. Jesus acknowledges the Father's position of authority when He says, "Everything is possible for you" and "if you are willing." *There is an element of correctly seeing that God has a place of authority, and it is to be rightly acknowledged.*

4. Jesus asks for what He wants. "Remove this cup from me," He asks. His "cup," His assignment, was always known. He was going to be the payment that sin requires for us to be brought back into relationship with Holy God. He was the "lamb of God" to be sacrificed so the debt of sin could be paid, and instead of death, humans could experience eternal life in the presence of God.[10] The assignment was not going to change, but I love in His human frame, Jesus shows angst over the reality of this assignment. *It is not a sin to ask, "Is there any other way?"*

5. The Garden of Gethsemane prayer ends for Jesus and also for us, when we are able to say, "Not my will, but yours be done." There is an element of not leaving the garden until we are able to leave our entire will there. Only then can you move forward in your assignment, carrying your cross to glorify God with a spirit of true biblical surrender. Because Jesus moved forward in His assignment and paid the sin penalty we ourselves deserved, we are allowed to have a direct relationship with God again.

The Bible promises that those who believe this and accept this gift of life will receive forgiveness of their sins, right relationship with God, and eternal life.[11] There wasn't really a question of whether Jesus was going to go through with His assignment to become the Deliverer for mankind. It had been the plan since the beginning of creation. But this Garden of Gethsemane prayer posture gives us the perfect form to emulate in our human frame as we walk through any assignment.

THE *heart* OF A BIRTH PLAN

EXAMINE BIRTH PLANS AND LORDSHIP: WHICH GARDEN IS IT?

The internet is full of different styles of birth plans. There are so many different templates and worksheets available for you to craft your ideal birth plan. Some hospital systems will even provide you with their own template you can fill in for all of your particular requests. Birth plans will outline desires for interventions, medications, positions, eating vs. not eating, IVs, monitoring wishes, pushing requests, perineal care, and baby care. You can customize a plan for environment lights, music, and I would even add what type of nurse you want for your birth. But can I tell you the truth? When I'm reading a birth plan, I am asking myself, "Who is Lord of this birth?"

Your birth plan and your own spirit will tell me. There is absolutely nothing wrong with asking for dim lights, limited medication, soft music, and position changes. There is nothing wrong about crafting an idea of your desired birthing environment and desired outcomes. There is nothing wrong with wanting a natural labor void of medication, limited interventions, and giving birth to a healthy baby without issue or incident. There is nothing wrong with that.

But what you will reveal to me is how tightly you are holding on to that plan. If you hold that plan loosely in your hand, flexible as labor shifts and changes, then you have released control and are on the road to surrender. But, friend, if you clutch that plan with two fisted hands close to your heart, you will show me you have a spirit of resistance and ultimately want to be Lord of your birth.

The word *Lord* used in the Bible has a Greek origin. The word is *kyrios*, which means "dominion, a power exerting itself in a particular jurisdiction."[12] You will need to decide who has dominion over your birth and who is in power. If you want to be Lord of your birth, I can tell you from experience it rarely goes that way. If the meaning behind your birth plan is to control and dominate and exercise Lordship, you may need to address the spiritual side of your birth plan.

Remember when I said to look at your birth plan, and I asked you, "Would you be okay if you didn't get ANY of those things, but you had a beautiful healthy baby?" What feelings did that invoke within you? Was there a feeling of panic? Was there an element of confusion? Did it arouse fear? If the thought of you not getting your ideal birth is NOT okay, then you are setting yourself up as Lord of your birth because you are grasping for control.

I assure you, whether the Bible is interesting to you or not, the notion of you as Lord of your labor will be challenged. These are spiritual questions that need spiritual answers. Birth balls and squat bars are not going to solve what is being revealed in your spirit. You will have to resolve who is Lord of your birth, spiritually. We have already established it is not nurses or doctors, so it is either you or a power other than you.

PREPARING A BIRTH PLAN WITH GOD AS LORD

If you are preparing a birth plan with God as Lord of your birth, it will look like a Garden of Gethsemane prayer posture. You can literally take any birth plan template from the internet and fill it in just as you wish. This is where we write everything we want and pour out our deepest heart desires. Asking for what we want is not bad or sinful at all. Go ahead and be as detailed as you want in this step. Write down everything you want.

THE *heart* OF A BIRTH PLAN

Next, literally give your birth plan to God and put Him in charge—as Lord. God wants to be in a relationship with you, personally. The goal here is to have a proper relationship with the Creator God to created man. If you need help or a reminder of who Creator God is, read Job 38–39. It will help you grasp how big God really is. Here is an excerpt:

―――――――― JOB ――――――――

"Where were you when I laid the earth's foundation?

Tell me, if you understand.

Who marked off its dimensions? Surely you know!

Who stretched a measuring line across it?

On what were its footings set,

or who laid its cornerstone—

while the morning stars sang together

and all the angels shouted for joy?

Who shut up the sea behind doors

when it burst forth from the womb,

when I made the clouds its garment

and wrapped it in thick darkness,

when I fixed limits for it

and set its doors and bars in place,

when I said, 'This far you may come and no farther;

here is where your proud waves halt'?

Have you ever given orders to the morning,

or shown the dawn its place,

that it might take the earth by the edges

> and shake the wicked out of it?
> The earth takes shape like clay under a seal;
> its features stand out like those of a garment.
> The wicked are denied their light,
> and their upraised arm is broken.
> Have you journeyed to the springs of the sea
> or walked in the recesses of the deep?
> Have the gates of death been shown to you?
> Have you seen the gates of the deepest darkness?
> Have you comprehended the vast expanses of the earth?
> Tell me, if you know all this."[13] | Job 38:4-18, NIV

I want to bring something into perspective for the church people; I had to learn this myself the hard way. But if I could share what I have learned in order to help you, I hope you will allow it. Asking for answers to a detailed prayer to a Holy God is never wrong. But sometimes, in our hearts we mean, "If You are God, show me by answering all my prayers exactly like this." Or "I know You will answer all my prayers, and I will praise you for it." Look deep into the prayer posture of these sentences. Who is really Lord in these heart attitudes? I hate to tell you. It's still you.

If you birth with these postures, you may be confused in postpartum as to why God didn't answer all your prayers exactly just so. I mean, after all, you believed Him for it. So why is it so faith shaking to pray and believe God for a certain birth and to end up with a different outcome? It is because you believed Him for His power but only wanted it in order to grant you what you held most dear. It's still you. It takes one to know one here, and I hope I can help you here because I did not understand this when I was praying for my own birth experience all those years ago. God is not there to give you three wishes or become your fairy Godmother. He really needs to be Lord. And if He is Lord, then you are not. Instead of asking God to grant you your will, giving God true Lordship is exchanging your will for His, no matter what the cost.

That's why the garden prayer is so important. It's here, in the garden, before your labor where you will take the first step in "taking up your cross." It's here. All the way back in the Garden of Gethsemane where you must deny yourself and crucify your own will to be ready to labor with God as Lord. You must deny yourself that which you want most. Your will, whatever your ideal birth looks like, needs to die. It actually needs to be crucified. It needs an ugly death, your will.

Dying to yourself spiritually is like watching spiritual sweat drops of blood falling to the ground as you feel the pain of dying to your own will. Dying to yourself is crucifying all your plans and desires. You're literally saying, "I intentionally am willing to deny myself what I want most (my plans of ____) in exchange for Your holy will, understanding that the cost may be great." This is biblical surrender when it comes to your birth plan.

Putting your birth story in God's hands will free you to "take up the cross" and go to your hospital birth. You will walk through the unknown of your birth with a renewed sense of relationship to Holy God as you become free to see God's plan for your birth and the gifts along the way. God wants a relationship with you. He is not always after answering all your prayers of comfort. Mercifully though, He does answer prayers of comfort, and there are many beautiful births and God-glorifying stories. But if His will is the hard road or the suffering path, can I just encourage you that you will be on a faith journey?

God has not forgotten about you but is drawing you closer. God wants you to trust Him and partner with Him in your assignment for His will and His glory. He may have plans for you that this birth may just be a small section of your overall story. He may not be done with your spiritual journey after your physical delivery, and a surrendered spirit will allow you to draw closer to God, even when you don't understand.

It is true Lordship to yield yourself to the plan and purpose of God. His ways are not our ways, and His thoughts are higher than our thoughts.[14] If we believe that, then we need the spiritual discipline of the Garden of Gethsemane in order to walk through the unknown. We need to first understand that God's plan for our lives as believers is we glorify Him on earth. We work together with Him to accomplish His plans and purposes for our lives. He doesn't promise we always know where it is going or how it's going to end.

All God ever expects from us is belief, and faith is truly all we ever bring—if we have faith enough to say in the garden, "Not my will, but yours be done." If we have faith enough to die to our own desires of comfort, Jesus will take us on the road to His glory. It may be full of ridicule, mocking, being made fun of, physical pain, relationship compromise, being hated, being alone, or giving up that which is most precious to us. That's what Jesus's carrying of the cross looked like. Be encouraged that our Savior Jesus walked the way of suffering before us. Now He walks it with us. We are never alone, and because of the presence of the Holy Spirit, we can pick up our crosses and endure our earthly assignments with a supernatural peace for a heavenly appointed purpose.

Your labor is no different. You must decide if you can spiritually emulate Jesus Christ in the Garden of Gethsemane, or will you take the path of Eve in the Garden of Eden? In which garden do you see yourself? Is it in Eden where Eve trusted the voice of her enemy, her own knowledge, and her own desire to be wise, all done while ignoring what God had already said? Are you wiser than God? Should He listen to you, or are you to listen to Him? Who is truly Lord?

The outline of the steps in the Garden of Gethsemane will lead to the path of a certain kind of righteousness that God loves. He loves submitted hearts and sweet surrender. It is in being honest with God about our human feelings during private prayer that we start to build a relationship with God independent of religion. It is personal. It is in correctly giving God His position of Lordship and submitting yourself to His all-knowing plan and purpose that a supernatural peace is found.

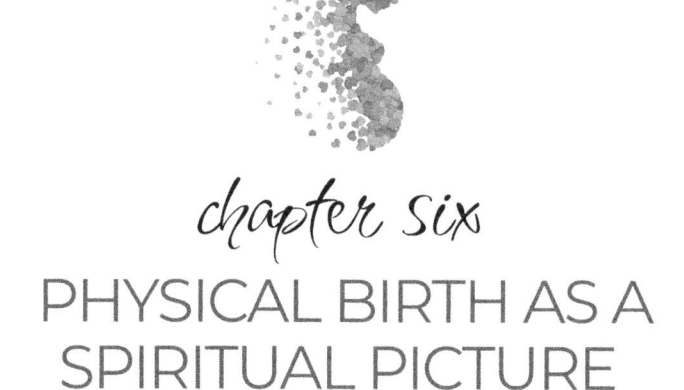

chapter six
PHYSICAL BIRTH AS A SPIRITUAL PICTURE

THE BETTER HOSPITAL BIRTH

You really can have a much better hospital birth experience by taking to heart the concepts of this book believing:

1. Your birth will be an assignment—it will unfold step by step, and you will have little control over your circumstances.

2. You give birth in a Genesis 3 environment—imperfect people, imperfect labor situations, where brokenness exists and undesirable variables to your birth can be a reality.

3. Your nurse is an expert in birth and Genesis 3 and can serve you greatly if you value her as a resource.

THE *heart* OF A BIRTH PLAN

4. You will have an element of pain—physical, emotional, or spiritual.

5. You will need to hone a spirit of surrender in order to partner with your nurse guide and perceive a positive birth experience.

But there's more.

God still uses the physical routines of our generation and time to illustrate spiritual concepts. One day as I was trying to help a laboring woman, I understood clearly there was a connection from labor and birth to our spiritual trials and tribulations on earth. This particular patient was completely resistant to any of my help and suggestions. Her labor was arrested (she stopped dilating), and she was in a lot of pain. Her labor turned from laboring to suffering, and I had some ideas as to how we could try some things to change her pattern and elicit some cervical progress.

But my suggestions went against her birth plan, and she would not let me partner with her in order to help her. I just seemed to stand by and watch her suffer until she was ready to accept advice or allow for a change. I wanted to partner with her, help her, and bond with her, but her spirit of resistance kept me at bay. Then it hit me!

That's me in that bed! I thought.

Not physically of course, but spiritually. I knew at the time in my own life God wanted me to write. But I was completely wrestling with Him about it and had every bit of the resistant spirit this patient was showing me. I literally was in tears over it, telling God why He completely had the wrong person, telling Him all the reasons why I couldn't do it and refusing to partner with Him in my new assignment. In fact, I was annoyed by it. There I was, interacting with actual authors God brought into my path, saying, "Look, God. Here's an author. See, she actually likes writing. Why don't you ask her to write?"

Having walked long enough with God to know the assignment doesn't change just because you don't like it, I was struggling with the faith it was going to take to obey in the journey. I was overwhelmed with the unchartered waters of trying to be a writer and truly never really even wanted to be one.

I was watching a patient being resistant to the idea of moving in a direction she didn't want to go in, refusing help, and being annoyed by my presence. It was a light-bulb moment for me! Similarly, here He was, the Great Physician at my spiritual bedside, trying to partner with me but ushering me into a different direction than I wanted to go. He wanted me to trust Him as He showed me the way.

But there I was, refusing the assignment with my resistant spirit. It was like I was saying spiritually what my patient was saying about her physical labor. "I know you're the expert, but I don't trust you because you are taking me where I do not want to go. This hurts, but I'm also afraid of where you will take me because it's new and not what I had planned."

Just like my patient, I was fearful of so many things. Resistant spirits cling to fear, and it is as true for life as it is for labor. I had to go to the garden to surrender my will, too, and it was a bloody crucifixion, my will. Crucifying fear and dying to self is required for walking in faith. I had to leave in the garden all my thoughts about what my family or coworkers would say about my writing and am continually laying down my fear of failure to walk in my assignment as a nurse writer. I wish I could tell you it was a clean process and a one-time thing. But for me, I can see fear and faith compete to occupy my thought life, and it is a continual battle of laying down my fears/wants/desires to walk with God and trust Him in my assignment.

PHYSICAL BIRTH AS A PICTURE OF SPIRITUAL BIRTH

I started paying attention to how else birth might be a physical picture of spiritual truths. It's amazing to me how something you can see with your eyes that repeats itself over and over all over the world can scream the most accurate picture of a profound spiritual truth. In fact, I would argue the most important spiritual truth of the whole Bible is spiritual rebirth.

Check this out. The actual act of physical birth.

In utero, a fetus is clearly alive but does not have to breathe on his own. His life is sustained by the umbilical cord connected to the mother's biology. The lungs are filled with fluid when inside the mother. It is at birth when the new baby must take his first breath of life. Once the umbilical cord is cut, the oxygen supply is cut, and this first breath of life must occur in order for the fetus to survive outside of the mother. The amazing part to me is the whole biology of the fetus is changed once this initial breath of life occurs.

With the first forceful breath, the breath of life physiologically forces air into the lungs and pushes the fluid out of the lungs. The lungs convert from fluid-filled sacs to air-exchange channels for the human body. That's why we like a good strong cry! It gets that fluid out of the lungs! When the first big breath occurs, lung expansion occurs, and lungs are cleared of this fluid and the body responds.

When the umbilical cord is cut, the blood pressure changes. Being detached from the life-sustaining placenta causes changes in the actual fetal human heart. The breathing and blood pressure changes of extra-uterine life (outside of mom's body) cause two shunts (or holes) in the heart to close. The baby starts a completely new cardiopulmonary system to sustain its life. The lungs change, and the heart itself is changed. The baby has a new way of receiving oxygen and circulating it, and it is very different from that which was in utero. This is the physical conversion that happens at the birth of every human baby.

At every birth, there is a picture of a physical conversion. This conversion to a new way of sustaining life is absolutely essential or the baby will die. In fact, when we learn how to resuscitate a baby, we learn that getting breaths in and ventilating a baby is the most important thing to do when trying to increase a heart rate that is too slow. If we can get good breaths in, this physical conversion will happen, and the heart rate will start to rise in response in most instances. The baby is unable to live outside the uterus without a new physiology. Old physiology cannot sustain the newborn. The baby will die without converting and changing.

The same concept is found in John 3 of the Bible when Jesus is talking to Nicodemus, who was a member of the Jewish governing body known as the Sanhedrin.

> Now there was a Pharisee, a man named Nicodemus who was a member of the Jewish ruling council. He came to Jesus at night and said, "Rabbi, we know that you are a teacher who has come from God. For no one could perform the signs you are doing if God were not with him."

Jesus replied, "Very truly I tell you, no one can see the kingdom of God unless they are born again."

"How can someone be born when they are old?" Nicodemus asked. "Surely they cannot enter a second time into their mother's womb to be born!"

Jesus answered, "Very truly I tell you, no one can enter the kingdom of God unless they are born of water and the Spirit. Flesh gives birth to flesh, but the Spirit gives birth to spirit. You should not be surprised at my saying, 'You must be born again.' The wind blows wherever it pleases. You hear its sound, but you cannot tell where it comes from or where it is going. So it is with everyone born of the Spirit."

"How can this be?" Nicodemus asked.

"You are Israel's teacher," said Jesus, "and do you not understand these things? Very truly I tell you, we speak of what we know, and we testify to what we have seen, but still you people do not accept our testimony. I have spoken to you of earthly things and you do not believe; how then will you believe if I speak of heavenly things? No one has ever gone into heaven except the one who came from heaven—the Son of Man. Just as Moses lifted up the snake in the wilderness, so the Son of Man must be lifted up, that everyone who believes may have eternal life in him."

> For God so loved the world that he gave his one and only Son, that whoever believes in him shall not perish but have eternal life.[1] | John 3:1-16, NIV

This beginning of John chapter 3 describes the core concept of the entire New Testament. Also, it reveals the promises of the Old Testament being fulfilled in Jesus Christ's life, death, and resurrection. God is doing a new thing. He is literally speaking to a religious leader, speaking to someone very precise in Bible knowledge, education, and experience in all things religion. But Jesus tells him a new thing.

That he must have a spiritual birth, a spiritual beginning where old ways are not enough, but he must become brand-new. He must have a spiritual conversion and be sustained by new physiology. The old physiology of "religion" must pass away, and the new physiology of "faith in Christ" will mark the start of a new spiritual life of repaired relationship with Holy God. You see, being stuck in Genesis 3 leaves us in our sinful state, and we have a fractured relationship with Holy God. We have to solve the problem that we are all sinners.[2]

Your spiritual birthday, your spiritual rebirth, comes when you understand Jesus paid the price you deserved for your sin.[3] You are literally set free from your own sin, and your very soul is purchased by the cost of Jesus's blood. He literally paid all you owe. If He died in your place personally, then He is your Savior, your Messiah. It is promised that whoever believes in Him shall not perish, but have eternal life.

When you are asked, "Who is Jesus to you?" it will require a response. It will be the same as that physical moment of a baby's delivery, where the cord is cut and old physiology is no longer valid. Religion cannot save you from your own sin. Following rules and being "a good person" will not be enough to solve the sin problem. We know this from the Nicodemus passage because Nicodemus was among the religious elite, yet he was told about needing to be "born again."

You may come to that spiritual crossroad where you will need to decide to breathe in a deep breath of faith and accept the spiritual gift of new life through the blood of Jesus Christ. Or you will say no, rejecting your spiritual birth, and the Bible says you will remain in an old physiology of religion that ultimately will lead to spiritual death.[4]

Spiritual rebirth is described much like the physical reality of newborn birth. If you "cut the cord" to your own methods of earning God's favor and accept the free gift of Jesus's death in your place, it will involve lungs and heart.

———————— ROMANS ————————

"For it is with your heart that you believe and are justified, and it is with your mouth that you profess your faith and are saved."[5] | Romans 10:10, NIV

You will use the breath in your lungs to confess with your mouth and literally call upon the name of the Lord.

———————— ROMANS ————————

"Everyone who calls on the name of the Lord will be saved."[6] | Romans 10:13, NIV

Your lungs have to literally cry out just like a newborn baby, and your spiritual heart needs to be changed.

EZEKIEL

> "I will give you a new heart and put a new spirit in you; I will remove from you your heart of stone and give you a heart of flesh. And I will put my Spirit in you and move you to follow my decrees and be careful to keep my laws."[7] | Ezekiel 36:26-27, NIV

A NEW CREATION

The Bible actually describes this spiritual conversion when you believe you are free from your sins as a birth of sorts and you become a child of God. As a child of God, all things will become new. You will have new desires and priorities, and old things will not seem as important to you anymore. "Therefore, if anyone is in Christ, he is a new creation. The old has passed away; behold, the new has come."[8]

The apostle Peter actually describes new believers as little babies. "Like newborn infants, long for the pure spiritual milk, that by it you may grow up into salvation—if indeed you have tasted that the Lord is good."[9]

There is a theme of growing as a believer in Christ and maturing as a Christian as you try to partner with God in faith moving through this life on earth. As a new creature in Christ, you will get new life circumstances or life assignments and what I have learned is the same concepts that apply to having a good hospital birth are the very same concepts that will help you spiritually as you try to walk with God here on earth.

1. You will get life situations you didn't ask for and maybe never wanted. I call them life's "labor" assignments. Everyone's assignments will look different. Some assignments might be a season, like a lost job or wayward teenager. Other assignments will be longer, like a cancer diagnosis or injury or marital problems. Some will be permanent for the rest of your earthly life. These may include disability, losing a husband or child, or bearing the scars of past abuses toward you. Whatever your earthly "labor" assignment, I assure you it will have a start and an end, even if the end is when Jesus returns or you breathe your last.

2. When your assignment starts, it will usually unveil itself as a piece of new information that will send you on a new journey. This journey will require faith in God as you move forward in it. God wants a relationship with you. Rarely does He tell you everything up front. You have to go through your journey step by step trusting Him for each day, and He will meet you in your assignment on the road as you are walking it. It will unfold piece by piece as God reveals until it ends.

3. Your assignment will take place in a Genesis 3 environment where suffering abounds, and sad outcomes are possible because of spiritual brokenness.

4. Just as you have a nurse as your "helper" in your physical labor and birth, in your spiritual labors on this earth, the Bible promises you a "Helper." If you are a new creature in Christ, the Bible promises the Holy Spirit is with you as your helper and to guide you.[10] Also, the Bible says Jesus Himself advocates for us in our situations.[11] Just like you can partner with your nurse for physical birth, our design as this new

creature in Christ is to use faith to trust in God and partner with Him in your assignment to glorify Him through it all.

5. Just like labor, we are promised an element of suffering and pain in our earthly assignments.

6. Coping with the pain and the totality of our earthly assignments will require surrendering of my own will as we understand Creator God is Lord, and He works all things for the good of those who trust in Him.[12] To truly live for Christ, you will move from labor resistance to surrender in your spirit and will be able to testify of the supernatural peace present with complete submission.

7. You may have an assignment in which you just may have to go to the garden before you can truly carry the cross. In your assignment, God may ask you to lay something down, and sometimes He asks you to lay down things that are so very important to you. It doesn't have to be sinful for God to ask you to lay it down. For example, if you have a sick loved one, praying for healing isn't sinful. But sometimes, healing is not God's will and you lose someone you love.

Remember, in the garden we can ask God for all the details of everything we want, but ultimately, we need to come to the place where you are okay sacrificing your will in exchange for God's and trusting Him for what you need as you move forward in your assignment.

8. God grows believers in Christ by asking them to exercise faith and to trust Him. Most of the time that means trusting Him when the earthly circumstances don't seem to make

any sense. There are many times in a believer's life when you will not see things clearly until many years later. Then you can see God-shaped footprints all over your story.

From Genesis to Revelation, the only thing continually commended by God is our faith. We let His glory shine when we don't understand in our human frame but trust Him anyway. I believe, and I think scripture supports this, that we will only be rewarded in heaven for the things we did on earth that required an element of faith in God to accomplish.

LOOKING FOR GOD'S GLORY IN MY LABOR STORY

Remember the younger girl described earlier in this book? It's the one with the natural birth plan, who took castor oil to beat her medical induction, who went into labor while the bridge was closed for road work, who ended up at the firehouse with a cute boy from high school being on duty, who ended up at the hospital for a million years, with every intervention, then a fractured coccyx, and a baby in the NICU? Remember her? Remember she sat in her postpartum room beating herself up and wondering, "Lord, this isn't what I had planned. Are You even there?"

Let me tell you how I see her now. I see a person who thought praying was coming to God with a list of things He was supposed to grant. She was a person who thought highly of herself and was very proud of her prehospital education. She thought she knew better than the medical people who had wanted to induce her a week before, but she refused. She refused because she had a resistant spirit governed by pride and fear. She was afraid of the medical community and thought they were her enemy. She doesn't remember her nurse because she was unable to bond with her. She carried false guilt into postpartum and thought she was weak and stupid. Maybe even her baby had to be in the hospital because of her foolishness.

Confused and hopeless, I was that person all those years ago. I had no idea why everything had to go so poorly. I didn't know how to see God in everything that had transpired. I had family and friends laugh at me because I was so far from a natural delivery, and I didn't even go to my birthing class reunion with all the other mothers because of shame. (That and my baby was still in the hospital.) I felt humiliated, physically in pain from my birth, and transitioning to life with a baby in the NICU.

My garden prayer before that birth was for God to grant me MY will. I wanted God to let me be Lord of my birth. I really wanted Him to grant my every desire. But the reason I wanted it was so I could show everyone how tough I could be (pride). Let me tell you, looking back on it, I can see God's protection over me, even as He corrected me as to who will be Lord in our relationship. Even though I was way off and my story is a great 3:00 a.m. story for all the labor nurses, through the years of telling it, I often leave out the parts of God's presence through the lesson.

That night, I believe running into the high school friend at the firehouse may have been the reason that the ambulance took me to my desired hospital instead of the closest hospital. If I had gone to the closest hospital, with the problems my baby had, he would have been transferred to a different level of care, and we would have been in two different places. To this day, I'm not sure if he had influence over this decision. But I am thankful I ended up delivering at a facility in which we were both recovering under the same roof.

Also that night, one of my bridesmaids, who was an NICU nurse, happened to be working at that hospital. I have a video of her presence in my delivery room looking after my baby, and I believe it was divine guidance that she was part of the team who cared for my baby. As a nurse now, when I look back on the atmosphere of my delivery, I can say I believe that God protected my son. With all the interventions and people in my room, I would bet on the fact that my baby probably didn't look that great on the monitor. Despite his delivery problems of meconium aspiration and eight days in the NICU, he had no ill effects from his delivery and is a smart kid, maybe too smart for his own good sometimes!

If you would have told me then I would become a labor and delivery nurse, I never would have believed you. It was years after this birth that I went to nursing school. I really felt like God was saying yes to this new move in my life. Going to nursing school was a team decision my husband and I made together, and it changed our lives and ended in a move for our family. It was a decision made to follow where I felt God was leading me, even though it wasn't a popular decision with some of my church friends or family at the time.

My nursing orientation on the labor unit, working with my amazing preceptor, was a healing time and a challenging time. Mentally I was learning so much, but I was also facing so much of what I had been afraid of during my own delivery. I was starting to really see how valuable a nurse can be in the medical birthing arena, and I wanted to do it well. I wanted to be a great advocate for patients, just like my preceptor.

Years later, God started weaving into my journey spiritual lessons along the way that happened to show itself at the bedside. Then, in recent years, I felt the push to write. Yes, at first I did wrestle. But honestly, as I just started walking forward in the assignment, it became clear why it couldn't be another writer. It had to be me because my story was crafted for it. It had to be the person who can identify with the resistant patient in the bed, who can see the different spirits of labor, and who can see the biblical parallels between physical labor and spiritual rebirth. I honestly feel that if my birth had gone the way I wanted it, I would not be suited to write this book. Reviewing my story now, I see how God's fingerprints are all over my story. What seemed so confusing at the time makes perfect sense now.

WHAT'S YOUR STORY?

I'm not sure of the circumstances surrounding your pregnancy. Maybe you are walking cautiously through an unwanted pregnancy, and choosing life is leaving you scared and unsure as you approach your labor and birth. Maybe you are trying to hold on to an IVF pregnancy and are wrestling with fear as you approach your birth.

Maybe this is not your first baby and you have done this many times and have picked up this book because you want it to be different this time around. Maybe you have just received a diagnosis with your provider at a regular scheduled appointment that has you concerned. Maybe you just wanted to see what a hospital nurse has to say about how to plan for a hospital delivery and had no idea this book would involve such a spiritual dynamic.

THE *heart* OF A BIRTH PLAN

Wherever your circumstances find you, I can promise you that if you embrace the heart of the matter when it comes to birth, you can see your birth story in a whole different light. Maybe your story will be just a simple birth and your assignment will be just that, a temporary walk through labor and pain that yields the glory of a new life. Or maybe your story will seem confusing to you when it is all said and done. In that case, maybe God is working on your heart in a new way that will be revealed later, as mine was. I just hope this book has helped you to open your heart to the possibility of your birth being a God story. He definitely is in the business of getting to the heart of the matter and drawing your heart closer to His as you trust Him to be Lord of your birth.

GOD'S NOT DONE

We have talked a lot about Genesis 3, so I feel it should be mentioned that God will not leave us in a Genesis 3 state forever. In the book of Revelation, His plans do have an end where He brings us to Himself in a place where no sin abounds. No brokenness, no pain, no suffering, no illness, and no death. But for now, we live in the time period known as the "church age." This is the time when salvation and eternal life is extended to any and all people. You don't have to know a certain religion or denomination to be accepted by God. We live in the earthly time period when anyone can be forgiven of their sins and will be promised eternal life through believing in Jesus Christ as their own personal Lord and Savior.

My heart for you is to have a wonderful hospital birth. I pray you would yield to your circumstances in your labor and bond with a wonderful nurse who will help you through it all. I pray for you to understand pain with progression and have a surrendered aura about you as you go through that which comes upon every laboring woman. I pray for your heart to be changed, softened, and renewed through your hospital birth experience and for you to walk out of the hospital with your healthy baby. I pray for God to show Himself Lord to your soul and to bestow upon you the peace that transcends all comprehension and it would guard your heart and mind through Christ Jesus.[13] Amen.

ABCs OF SALVATION
the physiology of spiritual rebirth

A | ADMIT YOU'RE A SINNER

Romans 3:10 "...None is righteous, no, not one"

Romans 3:23 "...for all have sinned and fall short of the glory of God"

Romans 6:23 "For the wages of sin is death, but the free gift of God is eternal life in Christ Jesus our Lord."

(Our old physiology will lead to death...we must cut the cord to religion and the efforts of 'trying to be good enough' to be with God)

B | BELIEVE JESUS IS LORD

Romans 10:9 "...because if you confess with your mouth that Jesus is Lord and believe in your heart that God raised him from the dead, you will be saved."

(Belief is the beginning of your new physiology!)

THE *heart* OF A BIRTH PLAN

C | CALL UPON HIS NAME

Romans 10:10 "For with the heart one believes and is justified, and with the mouth one confesses and is saved."

Romans 10:13 "For everyone who calls on the name of the Lord will be saved."

(This is your first heart's cry as a newborn of God...converting away from religion leading to death, and accepting Jesus as the way, the truth, and the life!)

John 14:6 "Jesus said to him, 'I am the way, and the truth, and the life. No one comes to the Father, except through me.'"

It will require your heart and your lungs!

Your spiritual rebirth begins with your change in heart and lungs just like a physical birth of a newborn baby! This calling upon Jesus is the proverbial "cry" of our souls to be saved from our sins and to walk in rebirth and newness of life. You can be forgiven, free, and have a personal relationship with God! You will use your heart and lungs to do it! Like a newborn, all things will become new!

2 Corinthians 5:17 "Therefore, if anyone is in Christ, he is a new creation. The old has passed away; behold the new has come."

The ABCs of Salvation are from JDFarag.org and are used with permission.

The ABCs amended for pregnancy and birth are the creation of Maria Maher and can be used by anyone for the purpose of sharing the gospel message for the salvation of souls.

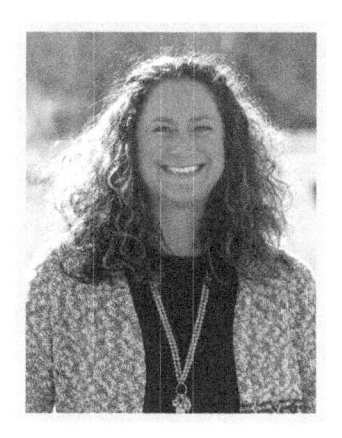

ABOUT THE AUTHOR

Maria Maher, BSN; RNC-EFM is an experienced registered nurse who has been working in the discipline of labor and delivery since 2009. Her passion is to help create sincere and productive conversations from a labor nurse to any prospective hospital birthing mother. She couples her experience at the bedside of laboring mothers with her heart to advocate for her patients in this writing, speaking honestly to expecting mothers.

Maria has been following Jesus since 2001 and is acutely aware of how life is a journey, and the spiritual journey, a progression. She writes from a biblical point of view as she highlights truths from labor, birth, and new life that aren't popular on the birthing videos, yet can make a difference in preparing a young mother for the hospital setting.

When she is not at the bedside, Maria is a wife to her husband of almost twenty years and has two sons. Maria is a doggie mom to an Aussie named Fenway who actually has a cameo in this book due to the lessons learned from her adoption and love found for a new breed!

ENDNOTES

CHAPTER ONE

1. "positive outcome." Medical Dictionary. 2009. Farlex and Partners 5 Jun. 2021 https://medical-dictionary.thefreedictionary.com/positive+outcome

CHAPTER TWO

1. National Academies of Sciences, Engineering, and Medicine; Health and Medicine Division; Division of Behavioral and Social Sciences and Education; Board on Children, Youth, and Families; Committee on Assessing Health Outcomes by Birth Settings; Backes EP, Scrimshaw SC, editors. Birth Settings in America: Outcomes, Quality, Access, and Choice. Washington (DC): National Academies Press (US); 2020 Feb 6. 2, Maternal and Newborn Care in the United States. Available from: https://www.ncbi.nlm.nih.gov/books/NBK555484/

2. https://admin.learningstream.com/files/DA1537B2-387C-452A-890E-A227518D8EB6_9/89605/03NICHD2008SummaryFetalMonitoringTerminology.pdf

3. www.dictionary.com/browse/control

4. https://psychologenie.com/insight-into-concept-of-normalcy-bias-in-psychology
5. Isaiah 46:9–10
6. Deuteronomy 31:6
7. Proverbs 3:5-6
8. Psalm 139:13–16

CHAPTER THREE

1. Wright, Christy, and Donald Miller. "Best The Christy Wright Show Podcasts: Most Downloaded Episodes." *Best The Christy Wright Show Podcasts | Most Downloaded Episodes*, 15 June 2021, www.owltail.com/podcast/28037-christy-wrights-business-boutique/best-episodes. BB Ep 2 Starting with the End in Mind with Donald Miller
2. "Breakdown of RN Nursing Requirements By State." *NurseJournal*, 29 Apr. 2021, nursejournal.org/registered-nursing/rn-licensing-requirements-by-state/.
3. Genesis 2
4. Genesis 3
5. Genesis 1:27
6. Genesis 1:28
7. Genesis 2:9
8. Genesis 2:17
9. Genesis 2:18
10. Genesis 2:25
11. Genesis 3:1

12. Genesis 3:4–5

13. Genesis 3:6

14. Genesis 3:7

15. Genesis 3:8

16. Genesis 3:10–13

17. Genesis 3:14–19

18. Genesis 3:22–23

19. Genesis 3:24

20. Romans 8:22

21. Romans 8:20–21

CHAPTER FOUR

1. Genesis 3:16
2. Galatians 6:7
3. https://www.dictionary.com/browse/deliverance
4. https://www.dictionary.com/browse/salvation
5. Micah 4:9–10
6. https://www.britannica.com/event/Babylonian-Captivity
7. Ezra 1:1
8. Genesis 3:17–19
9. Genesis 3:15
10. Isaiah 11:6–9

CHAPTER FIVE

1. Luke 9:23, NIV
2. Matthew 16:24, NIV
3. Mark 8:34, NIV
4. https://www.gotquestions.org/take-up-your-cross.html
5. Matthew 4:18–20
6. Mark 10:21–22, NIV
7. Matthew 26:36–39, NIV
8. Mark 14:32–36, NIV
9. Luke 22:39–44, NIV
10. 1 Peter 1:18–19
11. John 3:16–18
12. https://biblehub.com/greek/2963.htm
13. Job 38:4–18, NIV
14. Isaiah 55:9

CHAPTER SIX

1. John 3:1-16, NIV
2. Romans 3:23
3. Romans 5:8
4. Romans 6:23
5. Romans 10:10, NIV
6. Romans 10:13, NIV
7. Ezekiel 36:26-27, NIV

8. 2 Corinthians 5:17
9. 1 Peter 2:2-3
10. John 14:26
11. 1 John 2:1
12. Romans 8:28
13. Philippians 4:7

Made in the USA
Las Vegas, NV
30 January 2024

85124742R00095